THE CONCENTRIC METHOD IN THE DIAGNOSIS OF PSYCHONEUROTICS

Founded by C. K. Ogden

The International Library of Psychology

ABNORMAL AND CLINICAL PSYCHOLOGY
In 19 Volumes

THE CONCENTRIC METHOD IN THE DIAGNOSIS OF PSYCHONEUROTICS

M LAIGNEL-LAVASTINE

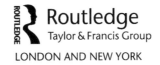

Routledge
Taylor & Francis Group

LONDON AND NEW YORK

First published in 1931 by
Routledge, Trench, Trubner & Co., Ltd.
2 Park Square, Milton Park, Abingdon, Oxfordshire OX14 4RN
711 Third Avenue, New York, NY 10017

First issued in paperback 2014

Routledge is an imprint of the Taylor and Francis Group, an informa business

British Library Cataloguing in Publication Data
A CIP catalogue record for this book
is available from the British Library

The Concentric Method in the Diagnosis of Psychoneurotics
ISBN 0415-20928-5
Abnormal and Clinical Psychology: 19 Volumes
ISBN 0415-21123-9
The International Library of Psychology: 204 Volumes
ISBN 0415-19132-7

ISBN 13: 978-1-138-88238-6 (pbk)
ISBN 13: 978-0-415-20928-1 (hbk)

CONTENTS

LIST OF ILLUSTRATIONS

PREFACE

LIFE flows towards its close—ever-quickening. The winged word lags behind the thought it expresses, and still more does the written word stumble on a thousand hindrances. The correction of a lecture once delivered has become a task I no longer willingly undertake.

Thanks to Mme. Chahine, who suggested that my lectures should be taken down by a stenographer and published just as they were, I offer to my colleagues these ten informal clinical lectures, as given by me in the beginning of 1927. You will find in them such faults as spring from extempore speaking; absence of bibliography, absence of a well-buffed and polished style, and of that didactic masonry that can bind a subject, in its entirety, into a strongly-knit, dogmatic structure.

I have, however, the somewhat simple hope that, as in certain literary notebooks, you may be able to distinguish a thought that, though fluid, is beginning to crystallize on contact with clinical realities. These lectures cover the diverse symptomatology of several clinical cases presented for study. I had originally wished, in six lectures given in my service at the Pitié, to demonstrate my everyday method of diagnosis of psychoneurotics. These six correspond to Chapters I, III, IV, VII, VIII and IX.

I have given to this volume the title of the third lecture, The Concentric Method in the Diagnosis of Psychoneurotics, for it is in the light of this personal method, which daily I find of the greatest service, that I have ordered and classified the clinical facts which I have presented. This method has the added merit of relegating to their proper place in the general biology the psychic facts, and of emphasizing that French clinical method, based as it is on morphological, physiological and psychological observation, can not, in the name of the clear and distinct ideas which guide it, allow itself to be led astray by certain psychometaphysical wanderings born of the work of Freud.

To these six basic lectures on the diagnosis of psychoneurotics, I have added four others, which complete and amplify them :

1. A lecture on Emotivity, which the "Association of Instruction of the Physicians and Surgeons of the Hospitals of Paris " asked me to give in the Hall of the old Academy of Medicine.

2. A lecture on *The Unconscious Self of Psychoneurotics in the light of Ascetic and Mystic Experience*, which is only an amplification of the lecture on Consciousness and the Unconscious Self of Psychoneurotics, which the recently formed Society La Maïeutique, that meets to discuss questions of the moment, asked me to give, with Baron Seillière, President of the Academy of Moral and Political Sciences, presiding.

3. A lecture on *The Devil in the Psychoneurotics*, which I asked my friend Jean Vinchon, assistant in my service, to make in remembrance of his excellent book, *The Devil*, which he wrote in collaboration with Maître Maurice Garçon.

4. Lastly, a closing lecture dedicated to *The General Principles in the Treatment of Psychoneurotics*, in reply to that constant criticism from the suffering public, that the doctor too often confines himself in his task to diagnosis, and to show that I have adopted as my own that banal saying of Alexandre Dumas fils, that no medical work is complete which does not bend all its forces to " sometimes cure, ease often, and always console."

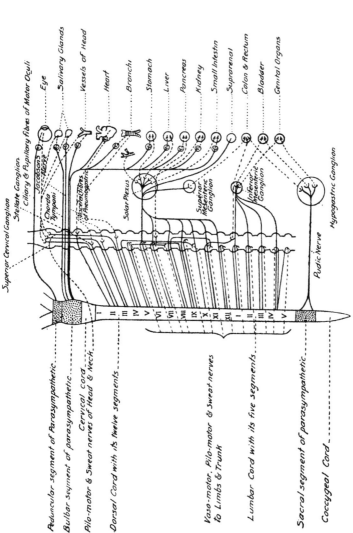

Fig. I.—Schema of the Sympathetic.

" Schema of the general distribution of the Sympathetic System, showing its division into vagal system (heavy black lines) and orthosympathetic, whose protoneurones are in fine black lines and deutoneurones in fine red dotted lines. The heavy dotted red lines indicate the deutoneurones of vagal character. The schema shows from left to right the medulla and cord, the sympathetic chain, the large ganglionic centres, the small peripheral visceral ganglia and the organ supplied. (After Cassirer and Pottinger, after Meyer and Gottlieb, after Eppinger, Hess, Falta, after Onuf and Collins, after Langley and François Franck.)"

The Concentric Method
in the Diagnosis of Psychoneurotics

I

DEFINITION AND CLASSIFICATION OF THE PSYCHONEUROSES

I AM beginning the year with six lectures on the practical diagnosis of the Psychoneuroses, and to-day I devote the first of these lectures to their definition and classification. First, a word of introduction—I am very fond of introductions, for they are occasions on which to play a little with general ideas. The idea underlying these lectures is this :

Alongside such sharply defined fields of scientific investigation as those of the various specialists—cardiologists, gastro-enterologists, dermatologists, psychiatrists, etc.—there are frontier regions, and for the past twenty-five years I have interested myself in their pathology. When I was an interne in a general medical service I interested myself in the psychic reactions of my patients When I became chief of service in hospitals, where my patients were mainly those suffering from nervous or mental complaints, I studied their visceral and humoral reactions, and it is my belief that there is no better way of convincing oneself of the necessity of always having this spirit of synthesis than the study of what one calls the psychoneuroses.

I shall go even further. The psychoneuroses not only have a relationship to medical questions, but also to literature, philosophy, religion and sociology. I believe then, that, to see clearly in a matter so complex, one must apply what I call the "shuttle method," not merely in the field of pathology but in the whole sphere of intellectual activity.

The " shuttle method " which I teach my students from their first days in a medical service, consists in going from the particular case, which they see in bed, to the general description which they find in books, and in going back again from the pathological description to the particular clinical case.

This method must be applied to cases of the psychoneuroses, and one must look for explanations of these conditions in the works of all authors dealing with such questions—in the mystic writers just as much as in the philosophers.

In such an investigation, the great fault to be avoided is the spirit of system. Distrust of the spirit of system is of great importance in studies which are still so little advanced as these are. Naturally one must have a hypothesis, a scaffolding on which to build, and in addition one must have a directing idea to enable one to group, at least provisionally, the various elements which one brings together. But it must be realized that the hypothesis is only the ribbon which serves to hold together, in a bouquet more or less well arranged, the different flowers, which are the collected clinical elements.

"Are we not an organized fantasy and is not our living being but a functioning incoherence and a disorder which acts ? Events, desires, ideas, do they not succeed each other within us in the most contrary and incomprehensible fashion ? What discords of cause and effect !" That phrase from *L'âme et la danse* serves as a text for what I have to say to you. That profound thinker, Paul Valéry, in digging down in the human soul lays bare this incoherence, this discord. One must not, therefore, be too precipitate in trying to illuminate it with Latin clarity : " Reason seems to me to be the faculty of our soul to understand nothing of our body," he says a little further on.

One must always keep contact with the *quid ignotum*. We must remain in the realm of facts and make as profound an analysis as is possible before passing on to synthesis, and this analysis must be made with various reagents ; it is the diversity of the reagents, that we shall use, that will enable us to penetrate the different layers of the psychoneurotics.

Such, then, is the general idea. I pass now to the practical side. I have told you that these six lectures were devoted to the practical study of the psychoneuroses, that is to say what the doctor must know in order to be able to orientate himself in the maze of didactic descriptions found in books.

Indeed, when in dealing with a case which appears difficult, the doctor who is not particularly *au courant* with the evolution of neuro-psychiatry refers to a book on the subject, he receives a very distinct surprise— descriptions by no means tally, the same things are described under different names, it is hard to know just where one is. It is here that the advantage of the oral lecture over the printed treatise lies, for in the former one can, as Bacon says, decant the matter so as to preserve only the essential facts.

Moreover, there is a period in people's lives when the instruction one gives them would appear to be, I believe, most profitable. Life, one might say, from the teaching point of view, is divisible into three periods : the first, in which one has a certain amount of leisure while not knowing yet a great deal from personal experience, one writes and consequently one's descriptions are chiefly secondhand, based on what one has read in previous authors. Then comes a period when, knowing things by personal experience, having lived them, one portrays them in the way in which one has understood them ; this period is not very long for, carried along by life's ever-quickening current, the time one can give to speculative research becomes more and more short, and soon one arrives at the third stage, in which things become stereotyped, in which one finishes, to some extent, by encysting oneself in formulæ, in which one begins to dream a more or less waking dream. One ends by no longer seeing reality save through ideas that have become crystallized in a brain of diminished plasticity.

It is my hope that I am still in the second stage, and I am taking the advantage of Time, which as you know is bald behind, to expose to you my conception of the diagnosis of the psychoneuroses or to be more exact the *diagnosis of the psychoneurotics*. To enable you to appreciate the difference between those two terms, I am going to bring several patients to your notice.

I. M.C.—This is a youth of twenty-four years of age, a grocer's assistant, who first came for advice last November. He walked with great difficulty on two crutches, because as he said he could not place a limb in a vertical position on account of pain. This patient represents the *cripple* type and he claims that his left lower extremity is useless. Now, examination of the most thorough kind has failed to demonstrate any objective sign at the level of the hip joint, in which he complained of pain, and there is complete absence of any physical sign of organic nervous system lesion. We gave him psychotherapy in the form of electrical current, and we were able to get him to leave without his crutches, and now he no longer uses them. But it is easily noticeable that he still has some doubt : for he is a doubter, is always timid, and is not yet completely convinced that he can do without a cane.

If we take the clinical-picture aspect of this case, we note the outstanding fact of a man who was convinced he couldn't walk, leave the out-patient room on a cane. This loss of function had been produced as the result of pain that he had had in the limb. There had been a process of auto-suggestion and in short we can say that he had a hysterical paralysis.

Here, then, is the first type of psychoneurosis: *Hysteria*. But it is unnecessary to go very much beyond this observation to see that, underneath this gross clinical manifestation of loss of function of the lower limb, that dominates the clinical picture, there is a mental state founded on doubt, fear, and loss of confidence in himself. We already see that in calling it hysteria we do not say very much; we put a label on the patient that refers to descriptions in books, but we are very well aware that there is much to be sought behind this label: we show up our own ignorance; and thus at least we already know something!

II.—This is the case of a woman, Mlle E——, who has come because she has had an attack of nerves about a month ago. She says that she began to cry; her legs gave way beneath her; she fell down, stiffened out, and showed well marked trembling; the attack lasted about twenty minutes. Forty minutes after she was better although she still felt depressed and sad.

Superficially, in the main, it is a hysterical or, as one calls it, an emotivo-pithiatic crisis. It is unnecessary to make any profound psychoanalysis to find an affective complex which has determined this nervous state, of which the hysterical attack is only a manifestation. Consequently, superficially, the rough episodic diagnosis is: hysterical attack.

On going a little deeper one finds: a psychic state dominated by a sexual idea or passion. Mlle E—— was in love with her brother-in-law; she represses this feeling; there is conflict and often the idea persists like an obsession. Here again we come on a very complex question.

Now, then, these first two cases, on which we put a diagnosis of hysteria, show up, when we go into them a little, the two great factors which one finds operative in hysterical people: *imaginative auto-suggestion* and an *emotive* cause, particularly when related to sexual manifestations.

III.—Here is a lady of fifty, who is pale and complains of headache. She says she feels blows on her head and neck ; she cries continually ; she complains of extreme fatigue. She has no digestive trouble ; on the contrary her appetite is very good. When one sees a pale woman of fifty who complains of headache the blood-pressure should always be taken, for very often such headache is associated with an early renal sclerosis, with hyper-tension. In the present case the blood-pressure is about normal, but there is present headache, asthenia, aprosexia (wandering attention), and rachialgia (pain in the spine). This is the clinical picture of *neurasthenia* ; consequently, the clinical label is : neurasthenia.

But one has not to go very far to recognize that this neurasthenia is not the first nervous manifestation in this woman. She had her first attack of neurasthenia when she was twenty-six ; she says that she became run down by overwork and hardship ; this attack lasted about two years. She had her menopause at a very early age, after a child she had and which she breast-fed too long. We have to do therefore with a *periodic depression* rather than with a neurasthenia : the prognosis is good.

Sometimes the diagnosis between renal sclerosis and the clinical picture of depression is difficult. But here it is undoubtedly a question of an intermittent periodic psychosis.

IV.—Here is a patient who has had a series of *phobias* since 1912 with periods of freedom. She has many troubles which vary with great rapidity ; thus she says that she has had uterine congestion, which would appear to have lasted three years during which time she was under treatment. Then when this was cured she says she suffered from a muco-membranous enterocolitis. A radiogram showed nothing. She claims to have been under treatment a further three years, when the condition was suddenly and completely recovered from. There-after she says she had hyperchlorhydria which disturbed her and gave her much pain ; she thought she had a cancer, lost weight and was afraid she had Addison's disease. Then suddenly the hyperchlorhydria got well. She next says she had " nervous bronchitis with rales " ; then from the bronchi the trouble went to her head ; she feared she might go violently insane, was afraid to use a razor, knife, or scissors ; she had them hidden away fearing that something stronger than herself might lead her to use them to kill her daughter or her grandmother. Her husband died in 1915 : mental shock. She was obliged to work and got well ; she got out of her morbid state.

Some time afterwards, the patient relapsed into this state of fear, fear of insanity, of killing her daughter or her grandmother whom she loves very much. Her grandmother died in 1921 : a fresh shock, and again an improvement occurred in her condition, she put on weight.

At the moment she is not depressed ; she is more agitated than depressed. Nevertheless she still thinks she has a nervous dyspepsia ; her pulse is very fast. She has no lesion, but she has a certain degree of over-activity of her sympathetic nervous system ; she is emotional and disturbed. That is why I always say to this type of case : " Every time you have an attack, ring me up," and I reassure them ; they are the sort of patients who must be reassured.

Here, then, is a patient who has a series of typical obsessions, which form the clinical picture of *psychasthenia*, and this is roughly the diagnostic label we put on her.

It is unnecessary to go very deep to realize that these phobias depend on two factors : one a *periodic state*, characterized by periods of depression, which have generally increased at the time of the shock ; and the other an *uneasy character*—of which the patient herself is aware— and in a way the increase in the periodic depression by the characteristic uneasiness has given rise to the typical manifestations, which come under the heading of psychasthenia.

V.—This is the case of another young female patient, that is extremely complex. She complains of having had curious attacks during which she had the impression that her life had become changed, that she was borne off somewhere else. She felt things which had taken place seven years previously ; she had the impression of living in another epoch—the *ecmnesia* of Pitres. She is highly emotional ; she shows marked instability of the vaso-motor system. Beyond this she shows a marked degree of visceroptosis, some slight scoliosis, and a somewhat unusual morphology.

Roughly speaking, she is an emotional case typifying the description, which we owe to Dupré, and which to-day is classical, of the Emotive Psychoneurosis. In analysing her thus summarily, one sees that in the course of her emotional crisis there are manifestations of the hysterical type : ecmnesia, the "supernatural state of infancy" described by Carré de Montgeron in the convulsionaries of Saint-Médard.

These several cases enable us in a way to schematize the four great varieties of the psychoneuroses : *Hysteria, Neurasthenia, Psychasthenia,* and *Emotive Psychoneurosis.* What then are the psychoneuroses ? What is the defi-nition ? I am not going into the historical aspect : nor shall I give a definition "*per genus proximum et differ-entiam propriam*" in the manner of the Logic of Port-Royal. I shall simply make an arbitrary division of the facts. I do not want so much to speak to you of the psychoneuroses as of the psychoneurotics. These patients I have just shown you are psychoneurotics. How are we to distinguish them from the other patients in the clinic ?

To do this we must establish two limits : first a limit on the neurological side, then a limit on the psychiatric side.

On the neurological side the limit is demarcated by all the syndromes which are accompanied by physical signs of organic lesion of the nervous system, according to the criterion of Babinski, at the same time keeping in mind that there is, often enough, association between the psychoneuroses and organic nervous affections.

On the psychiatric side the limit is equally easy of determination from the big psychopathic syndromes, characterized as they are by the subject's unconsciousness of the situation and his conduct determined as it is by pathological urges and motives.

One eliminates then, from the start, all the big hallucinatory psychoses, whether systematized or not, the psychoses of interpretation, of revindication, and all the psychoses of organic origin having physical signs of organic nervous lesion.

This limitation, however, on the neurological and psychiatric sides is not enough ; one must " rewash " as in chemical analytical procedure.

Let us " rewash " first on the nervous side : From the time of Charcot, who had a schematic mind which rendered the greatest service in the establishment of neurology, onwards, the matter was simple ; in one group one placed organic nervous affections with physical signs, and in another the remainder, forming the vast group of functional manifestations, of which the type was hysteria.

But in this so-called functional group, it was realized very soon, there were a certain number of manifestations, which, while perhaps they could not be correlated with lesions, detectable by our methods of investigation of the moment, were yet not the consequence of a simple psychic trouble. In other words there are *functional manifestations which are not psychogenetic*. And it was thanks to Babinski that they were brought together under the heading of *physiopathic* symptoms, which he opposes to organopathic syndromes due to detectable lesions. It is this physiopathic syndrome which we have seen so often during the war, and the reflex paralysis, described by Vulpian, belongs to this type.

A certain number of affections, such as epilepsy, also belong to the physiopathic syndromes, since there is often, during or after an attack, extension of the great toe on the metatarsal bone, which is a sign of disturbed function of the pyramidal system. These physiopathic syndromes, which show the signs not of lesional organic disturbance but of dynamic organic disturbance, are *dynamic non-psychogenic nervous syndromes.*

On the mental aspect the situation is similar, we have to note light, attenuated, forms of the main classical psychopathies : slight delusional insanity, psychotic sense of being wronged, passion psychoses, in which there is still a relative consciousness of the social situation, and which do not end in such reactions as demand certification.

Equally there exist attenuated forms of melancholia which may alternate with periods of excitement,which have been described under the name of *conscious melancholia.*

On the mental side then may be included psychoses similar to those described above, but they are attenuated forms, such as I describe as " button " psychoses, and which one cannot diagnose unless one has lived for a long time with the classical psychopaths that one finds in the Insane Institutions, for their manifestations are often, in daily life, very attenuated, and in a way one must know how to recognize the grand ceremonial costume in order to be able to differentiate it from the modest garb of everyday wear.

In these " button " psychoses, then, there is in the first place a relative consciousness of the pathological characters of the manifestations, and, in the second place, a relatively possible social behaviour arising from the fact that the individual does not yield to the pathological urges.

I believe, by this double limitation, that I have shown you the region in which psychoneurotics are evolved. The psychoneuroses are not diseases ; neither are they affections, nor are they syndromes : they are merely *evolution moments of neuro-psychiatric syndromes.* And to make a diagnosis, in general, I recall to your mind the sieve that must always be used to sift complex cases.

In general medicine, the first diagnosis is that of the *syndrome*, that is to say the clinical signs which are the expression of a disturbance of function ; next one passes to the diagnosis of the *affection*, that is to say the morbid site of the disease. The diagnosis of the *disease* is then made by bringing together the signs which enable one to correlate the case under study either with an infection, intoxication, tumour, or vitamin deficiency, etc. : thus the ordinary diagnosis is made.

In psychiatry, there is an additional diagnosis, which I have termed the " *clinical picture diagnosis*," which is determined by the patient's reactions, which may be melancholic, megalomaniac, ideas of persecution, etc.

Let us see what the standards are that allow us to recognize that we are dealing with the psychoneuroses. There are two : one neurological, the other psychiatric.

Neurological criterion.—It is first of all a *negative standard* : absence of physical signs of organic affection of the sensory-motor nervous system, no inequality of the tendon reflexes, no disturbed sensation.

Then there is a *positive criterion* : objective signs of dynamic nervous disturbances in the field of the sympathetic.

Psychiatric criterion.—Here again there is a double criterion, negative and positive.

Negative criterion.—There is present neither unconsciousness of the situation, nor behaviour determined by pathological urges or motives.

Positive criterion.—First, there is a certain domination of the conscious by the unconscious. In the second place one notes a dominance of the sympathetic over the cerebro-spinal system. One might say that they are people who are not completely awake ; their complete differentiation between waking and sleeping, between perfectly rational life and their unconscious is not absolute ; they are people in whom sympathetic reactions are predominant.

This diminished differentiation in functions, this lowering of faculties of the higher order to the inferior sphere are the expression of regression towards the primitive phase, the infantile phase ; this is why, very often, we find in psychoneurotics psychic manifestations found in primitive races, and which have been so well described and analysed in Levy-Bruhl's publications.

Classification.—Such then, roughly, are the characteristics found in psychoneurotics. How shall we classify these psychoneurotics ? Shall we keep the classical grouping ? I am prepared to keep it, as an Ariadne's thread, to guide us in the labyrinth of the psychoneuroses; and, following the reaction-features which strike the ordinary person, I am willing to keep the didactic division of the psychoneuroses as : *Hysteria, Neurasthenia, Psychasthenia,* and *Emotive Psychoneurosis.*

Hysteria is characterized by manifestations, resembling many ordinary affections, which can be perfectly reproduced by the will and can be made to disappear under the influence of persuasion alone. This is M. Babinski's definition of *pithiatism.* It is purely a clinical symptomatic division, and we shall say that hysteria is present whenever we find these important features of the primitive manifestations of hysteria reproduceable with sufficient exactitude by the will and capable of being caused to disappear by persuasion. The secondary manifestations of hysteria are those which follow the primary.

Pithiatism, which is a definite syndrome, does not exhaust the psychological riches of the hysterical. On digging down a little one sees that there are processes of auto or hetero-suggestion, a product of overfull imaginations, which often end in delusional manifestations. One might even have said that hysteria was the psychoplastic form of delusion.

On the other hand, these manifestations are often the outcome of emotions of relative intensity often connected with worries, shocks, or sex emotions.

Neurasthenia is a syndrome described by Beard in 1880,

and is characterized by asthenia, cephalalgia, rachialgia and aprosexia, and a facility for auto-suggestion from the fact that the individual is preoccupied with the state of his health. At the same time, there is often a certain degree of sadness, digestive troubles, and vascular variations characterized by at one time hypertension at another hypotension. But the thing which characterizes neurasthenia above all is the state of *fatigue*.

We shall see that this syndrome in the pure state is extremely rare and that the greater part of the time it is only a stage in the development of the manifestations of a periodic psychosis.

Psychasthenia has been described by Janet. It is a synthetic condition, in which he grouped, on the one hand, the " obsessed " of the psychiatrists and, on the other, a certain number of constitutional asthenics. He has shown that these paroxysmal syndromes of the psychiatrists, characterized by obsession, appeared on a background which was itself characterized by a diminution of the " élan vital." The patient has the impression that he is in a dream. We shall see that in analysing these psychasthenics one notices that the thing which characterizes them is doubt and anxiety : *anxious doubt*.

Finally, *Emotive Psychoneurosis* is the association of the persistence of infantile emotivity, which may be increased by the influence of certain affections, shocks or repeated emotions as in the war, for example, and the enormous facility of sympathetic reactions in proportion to the emotions felt—reactions, may one say, which are quite discordant. The characteristic then of the emotive psychoneurosis is the disequilibration resulting from emotion, this exaggerated emotion being very closely connected with the functioning of the instincts, in such a way that one may say that this excessive emotion is a " *misfire* " of instinct.

In these four main types hysteria, neurasthenia,

psychasthenia, and emotive psychoneurosis, we find, then, essentially, a disturbance of imagination, fatigue, anxious doubt and various emotions.

The *conclusion* to draw from this first lecture is that, in the present state of neurology, these four divisions of the psychoneuroses must not be preserved in the study of the somatic manifestations which accompany them. They will still serve us as a landmark, but I shall show you that there is an association of these conditions in a way that one might almost call constant. As early as in the time of Charcot they spoke of hystero-neurasthenia. The last case I showed you has features of neurasthenia, hysteria, psychasthenia, and emotive psychoneurosis.

There is, then, a need to replace this fragmentary, superficial, symptomatic diagnosis, of the surface, which one has made up till now, by what I call the " *diagnosis in depth.*" I shall show you in the next lecture that in applying the concentric method in the diagnosis of the psychoneurotics, one comes to understand the patients infinitely better and consequently to have better methods of treating them. For, after all, the objective we ought always to have in view is not an ideological promenade in the gardens of pathology, but a patient search to find the best possible way to ease suffering humanity.

II

EMOTIVITY

My first word is one of thanks to the initiators of these Sunday lectures, and to an audience which is good enough to do me the honour of coming to work even though it be a day of rest.

I am going to bring before you Emotivity, a subject which is a world in itself, for the emotional are legion. I shall try to be as concise as possible, so as not—as far as is in my power—to overstep the hour allotted to me.

Emotion is a complex psycho-organic phenomenon, resulting from a sudden change in the conditions of adaptation of the affective tone of the tendencies.

That is the definition of the *emotion-shock*, which is the first stage and which is next followed by the *emotion-feeling*.

This definition of emotion distinguishes it from the *passions*, such as one understands them to-day, and from this point of view I must give you the modern definition, which is not the same as you will find, for example, in Descartes, in his " Treatise on the Passions," or in the old psychology.

Formerly, one understood by " passion " what one calls to-day "emotion"; whereas the passions, in modern psychology, are the inherent or acquired tendencies, which derive from other tendencies, group themselves, impose themselves, and become the attraction centre of all the feelings and tend towards realization.

As a consequence passion is a *chronic organized affective state*, and is much more developed as a psychic process than the emotive process You see that my definition

15

of emotion goes much farther than that which you may still find in Taine's psychology.

Taine had the merit of shedding much light on psychological phenomena, but he was too arbitrary in his conceptions, and in his psychology emotion appeared to be an elementary factor, in a way the unit of the affective sphere, as sensation is the unit of the representative sphere. But it is very evident that all psychological phenomena have each a representative charge, both affective and motor, and it is only a predominance of one or other in the charge that determines the nature of the manifestations of the moment.

On the other hand, it was the great merit of William James, in America, and Bergson, in France, that they showed that we were constantly carried away while emotion was operative, that our psychology was but a moving wave of manifestations which are never the same, and that what discursive intelligence does, in trying to establish categories in such things, is never anything but an arbitrary outlining, useful in practice, but in no way corresponding to the deeply underlying reality.

This is why I consider emotion—as I said to you—as a *complex psycho-physiological phenomenon resulting from a sudden change in the conditions of adaptation of the affective tone of the tendencies.*

We are essentially tendencies ; every creature, by the mere fact of his existence, tends to continue in his being, according to Spinoza's principle. These tendencies are varied according to their origin and purpose. You are aware that Pierre Janet divides them essentially into three great categories : the *lower tendencies*, of visceral origin, which have a precise somatic source and give rise to the bodily needs ; the *superior tendencies*, whose origin, on the contrary, cannot be localized exactly in the body, and whose trend is towards synthetic functions of a superior order, social, religious, æsthetic ; and the *intermediate tendencies*, which are characterized, on the one hand, by their starting point being still in the organ-

ism, and, on the other, by having their end point in the
more or less elevated parts of the psychic sphere.

There would be, then, emotions in all these varieties
of tendencies, these emotions being themselves more or
less elevated, more or less idealized, according to whichever tendencies they accompany.

Some people have wanted to say that all the emotions
were the expression of an instinct. I believe that is going
too far. On the contrary, one can say that all the instincts
have always an emotive side, but the tendencies do not
amount to the same thing as the instincts. There are
some that are characterized by *needs*, others by *desires*
and others again by *tastes*. And in each of these,
cases one always finds an emotive element.

If now we schematize the question and fix our attention
on definite points, to better delimit our subject, we see
that the emotions group themselves essentially round four
fundamentals : pleasure, pain, fear and rage.

I am going to say a word about the *emotions*, to analyse
their elements, then I shall go on to *emotivity*, also to
distinguish its elements ; I shall thus have an *analytic
study* which will allow me subsequently to construct a
synthesis of emotivity, from which I shall draw several
practical and *theoretical conclusions*.

Now, emotion has *two aspects* : the *psychological aspect*
and the *organic aspect* ; on that point everyone is in
agreement. It is a *psycho-somatic complex*. Also, emotion
has *two stages* : the first, the *emotion-shock* ; and the
second, the *emotion-feeling*.

When individuals are perfectly adapted to their
environment and their tendencies find their logical outlet
in the material, representative or social surroundings,
there occurs only such slight variations in their affective
tone that the emotion-shock does not occur.

But this is not the rule, and more usually emotion is
accompanied by a little shock, a little jolt. This is the
emotion-shock, characterized, as I told you, by a *psychic
element* and, also, by a *visceral disturbance*.

C

Let us look at these two elements in the four great categories.

In *pleasure*, you are familiar with the affective tone, the somatic manifestations which accompany it, the tendency to straighten up, the increase in muscular tone, the tendency to vaso-dilatation, and an impression of increase in will power.

On the other hand, in *pain*, from the somatic point of view, there is the tendency to be bowed down, vaso-constriction, and diminution in muscular tone, only however when the pain is not severe enough to produce a compensatory reaction, for *there are pains which are dynamogenic*.

Fear, which, one may say, is the defence manifestation of the instinct of self-preservation, is characterized, psychically by a very painful emotion and, somatically, by two orders of manifestations, according to whether one is dealing with passive or active fear. *Active fear* is characterized muscularly by flight, by the somatic reactions affecting the sympathetic, and even by secretory manifestations which may go very far, as various expressions in the vocabulary you know indicate. On the other hand, the *inhibitory form* may terminate in an actual paralysis of the different functions ; inability to stir. The individual is nailed to the ground, or even sometimes he has the feeling that his limbs give way under him, and in this we have the possibility of hysterical manifestations appearing under the influence of fear.

I had a remarkable example of this a few years ago, in my Laennec service. It was the case of a servant, who so loved her mistress—a rare thing to-day—that when the latter fell into a pond, the servant in presence of this dramatic spectacle, lost her speech and collapsed, losing the use of her legs. She remained in this state, dumb and paralysed, during ten years, in spite of several hundred injections and the visits of several dozens of doctors. She came into my service with the greatest of difficulty as she was a provincial. In one day I gave her back her speech, and in two days she walked. She then returned to her home, where the local inhabitants turned out to meet her ; and they put up in the middle of the town a fine triumphal arch with " Honour to my Saviour " on it. There is a remarkable example of hysterical manifestations following on fright.

Next, *rage* : rage is the aggressive form of the instinct of self-preservation that has received a jolt. The animal form of rage is aggression : an angry cat attacks a dog, scratches it, etc. The human form may be an aggression reduced to a few muscular movements, and thus an angry man relieves himself by waving his arms, stamping his feet, giving vent to exclamations, or breaking something. A much higher degree of civilization is necessary to act like M. Bergeret, who, surprising his wife in a much too intimate conversation with M. Roux, contented himself in a dignified manner by taking up from a table a copy of the *Revue des Deux-Mondes*. But I believe that this absence of reaction is a physiological mistake. For in so doing, this good M. Bergeret diverted to his sympathetic nervous system the nervous influx, which he should have worked off normally on his striped muscular system, and he must have suffered for some time the manifestations due to this displacement.

Be that as it may, such are the chief gross manifestations of the four fundamental emotions : pleasure, pain, fear, rage.

But, after the visceral disturbances of these emotion-shocks, a state of relative relief is established, which is characterized by the *emotion-sentiment*. Many emotions have a very slight emotion-shock, and are chiefly developed in the emotion-sentiment. Such is the case with the emotion of tenderness, on which I should have to dwell at length, only I do not care to do so, for thus I should touch the confines of love . . . and you know that it is infinite !

In this field of tender emotion one may have emotion-shocks : there is the *thunderbolt* of love at first sight, as well as manifestations connected with the genital and social instincts. I need not stress this more.

I merely want to emphasize amongst these rapidly made first statements the necessity of making a fuller analysis of the different elements, which one finds in emotion, and I suggest that we arrange these under three headings : first, a *psychic element*; second, the *expression of the emotion* : and, third, the *somatic concomitants*.

I shall pass over the psychic element very quickly. What I want remembered is simply that the instincts, the tendencies, have always an emotional aspect, and that there is a very distinct parallelism between the facility of the emotions and the predominance of the instincts in the psychic field. If, for example, one follows the evolution of human psychology, from birth to death, at first the instincts are dominant, because the higher synthetic faculties are not yet developed. This is the chief period of emotivity.   In the autumn and winter of life, there is a tendency for the higher faculties to go to sleep ; there is reappearance of instinctive predominances, the appearance of senile emotivity.   There is, then, a very distinct relationship between the two and this explains why a very distinguished author humorously gave this definition of emotion : " It is a misfire of instinct."

I pass now to the *expression of the emotion*. This can be studied, in the first place, in the countenance : it consists of the study of *facial expression*, so much used by Darwin and by Duchenne of Boulogne, and, also, the study of the general expression of the individual, with his attitude and bearing—his behavior, as the Americans call it.

I do not lay stress on modifications of *tone in striped muscle* ; I merely want to recall to you that there is no proportional relationship between the intensity of emotive expression and the depth of affective tone.   There is often, indeed, a relationship in inverse proportion. " Still waters run deep."

I come now to the third element : the *concomitant somatic element.* The constancy, during emotion-shocks, of somatic manifestations particularly affecting the sympathetic field has long been noted. In the most general way these are vasomotor reactions, unstriped-muscle contractions, (intestinal or pulmonary), and secretory reactions ; in short, modifications in the general metabolism which result in changes in the body fluids. I have otherwise studied these sympathetic reactions and from the practical standpoint I separate the cases examined, according to the responses of the oculo-cardiac and solar reflexes, into four main reaction-types : the *pure vagotonics,* in whom the oculo-cardiac reflex alone is exaggerated, the *ortho-sympathicotonics,*[1] in whom the

[1] In the introduction to his *Pathologie du Sympathique,* Prof. Laignel-Lavastine clearly defines his terminology :

" I therefore call the *Sympathetic,* or *Vegetative,* or *Autonomic System,* the whole nervous system which regulates the functions of nutrition, in the widest sense, or, better, the system regulating those functions, which are not voluntary sensory-motor functions. Going back to Winslow's terms I call the *great sympathetic,* the sympathetic of Langley, whose efferent protoneurones are derived from the thoraco-lumbar cord.

" I call *lesser sympathetic* or *vagal system* the *parasympathetic* of Langley including the *vegetative part of the pneumogastric* or *bulbar parasympathetic* and the *pudic* or *pelvic parasympathetic.*

" Langley emphasized the chiefly visceral rôle of the parasympathetic in relation to the general nutritional rôle of the orthosympathetic. The general plan of the autonomic system, says Langley, lies in the fact that the sympathetic sends its fibres into every part of the body, while the bulbar, tectal and sacral systems send their fibres only into special regions.

" Gaskell repeats the same idea in saying that the great sympathetic is more a system of vegetative life whereas the organic life is in the field of the parasympathetic. This explains why fibres of the orthosympathetic go to the cranial and pelvic territories of the parasympathetic.

" This same idea has been taken up by Cannon.

" The efferent fibres of the two parasympathetic systems, says Cannon, differ typically from those of the thoraco-lumbar part in having but few of the characteristic diffuse connections of the latter and in innervating separately the organs to which they are attributed. The preganglionic fibres of the cranial and pelvic systems thus resemble the nerves of voluntary muscles, and their arrangement provides for similar possibilities of separate and specific action, in no matter what part, without action occurring in the other parts.

" Finally, I call *small sympathetic* what remains of the parasympathetic after the elimination of the vagus and the pudic, that is to say the vegetative elements of the *motor oculi* (*ocular or tectal parasympathetic*), of *the pars intermedia of Wrisberg* (*chorda tympani*) and of the *glossopharyngeal* (*Jacobson's nerve*). It is to be noted here that the trigeminal,

solar reflex alone is exaggerated, the *hyper-orthosympathi-cotonics*, in whom the oculo-cardiac reflex and the solar reflex are exaggerated, and the *hypo-sympathicotonics*, in whom these same reflexes are elicited with less response than in those subjects in whom the variations may be considered as swinging within normal limits.

To come back to the *somatic concomitants* of emotion. These have received much attention from the Anglo-Saxon authors and particularly from Lange, who had noted the vaso-motor variations, the changes in muscular tonus, the secretory manifestations, and who believed he could make a true discrimination between the different emotions according to the sympathetic disturbances noted.

Thus he said : " *Disappointment* is a function of diminished muscular tone, and if to this be added vaso-constriction *sadness* is produced. If to this diminished muscular tone with vaso-constriction is added organic spasms, we get *fear*. On the other hand, if there is, with the diminished muscular tone, simply inco-ordination of visceral reactions, *embarrassment* results. If, to the opposite condition, increased muscular tone, there is added organic spasms ? *Impatience*. And to increased muscular tone, if vaso-dilatation is added, *joy* is produced. On the other hand, if, to increased muscular tone and vaso-dilatation, inco-ordination is added? *Rage* results ! "

It is too pretty and too simple. It had, however, a great vogue : it constituted the *vaso-motor theory of Lange*, which in the first place is quite wrong in reducing the concomitant sympathetic reactions to simple vaso-motor

---

which has close connections with the ophthalmic, spheno-palatine, and otic sympathetic ganglia, has no motor nucleus which gives rise to vegetative efferent protoneurones.

" And as conciseness is one of the good qualities of speech, I also call the sympathetic system in its entirety : *Holosympathetic* (ὅλος entire), the holosympathetic being divisible into the *great sympathetic* or *orthosympathetic* (ὀρθός straight), and *parasympathetic* (παρά along-side) corresponding to the sense in which it is used by Langley. I prefer the term parasympathetic, chosen and consecrated to Langley, to that of *symvagus* (σύν with), which was proposed by Sicard to designate the same parts of the holosympathetic, which are neither the thoraco-lumbar sympathetic nor the local visceral systems."—*Trans.*

reactions ; *the vaso-motor is not the whole sympathetic effect.* And, in the second place, it is wrong in that, in a way, it only deals with what is the contrary and only a part of the emotive manifestations.

Nevertheless, the philosopher William James was so taken with the inductions of Lange that he formulated his famous theory, which they are still teaching in the secondary schools, to the joy of the school boys, and which, if you care, can be expressed in the three phases : " I am grieved, because I am crying ; I am annoyed, because I strike ; I am afraid, because I am trembling." But the great English experimental physiologist Sherrington took a dog and divided its spinal cord in the lower cervical region, leaving intact the connections with the sympathetic system, and he studied the emotive reactions of this dog, which, be it noted, was separated from all the lower part of its body, except that it had the sympathetic connections. And those reactions remained those of a normal dog. Next, in this same animal, he cut the cervical sympathetic, in order to isolate the brain from the rest of the body : the dog continued to have the reactions of fear and rage of a normal dog. But Lloyd Morgan raised this objection, he said: " Your dog still has its memory, and consequently memory associations allow emotive reactions in the cephalic extremity, without the animal having, of necessity, true emotive complexes." To which Sherrington answered : " These operations were done on an animal nine weeks old, an age when it has not yet acquired all its affective equipment." Consequently Sherrington's observations are of great importance and show that William James's theory does not fit the true state of affairs. It is incomplete.

You see the importance of the somatic concomitants. Those Anglo-Saxon authors have gone too far ; but that is no reason, because they have tried to explain everything by the physiological manifestations, why one should deny the rôle played by these ; it is merely a question of getting things in their proper place.

But there is something else besides the manifestations of unstriped muscle contraction and the vaso-motor ones that I have already mentioned. There are most important secretory manifestations. These have been very fully studied by Pavlov, and in this connection we shall bring in, in its proper place, the phenomenon of consciousness.

Everyone knows of Pavlov's work on the dog, with a gastric fistula, which enabled him to study these secretory reactions. If food be placed in the stomach through the fistulous opening, without the dog having seen it, a scanty secretion of gastric juice follows, which is due to the direct stimulation of the stomach by the food in question. If, on the other hand, one shows the dog a favourite food, without allowing him to eat it, the mere sight of it will cause the secretion of a *psychical juice*, which is infinitely more rich in digestive qualities than the juice first secreted. Now, in the first case, there was a reflex whose starting point was purely locally somatic, in the second case, there entered the phenomenon of consciousness, which consisted in the desire to eat an appetizing thing that the animal saw.

This shows you the wisdom of the worthy Brillat-Savarin, who was both a good psychologist and psycho-physiologist, and whom Medicine must heartily admire ; and, on the contrary, how wrong is de Musset's line : " Qu'importe le flacon, pourvu qu'on ait l'ivresse !" (" What matters the wine, so long as one has the ecstasy.") He must have been of a somewhat callow youthfulness to write that ! The importance of gastronomy is evident.

Further, the secretory reactions must be studied in their various relationships, and *emotion* is a *reaction* of *poly-motivity* as it is also in a way a *poly-glandular* reaction. The secretory reactions are not only external ; they are also internal. The external reactions have been very fully studied by my two friends, Prof. Georges Dumas and Prof. Maloisel, who, in connection with his thesis on the salivary glands, investigated the reactions of these glands during emotions.

All glands secrete in ways varying according to the emotions ; and such glandular reaction applies not only to the glands of external secretion but also to the endocrine glands. And these endocrine secretions vary. Cannon has laid much stress on the importance of this. He noted that people who attend sporting events, such as at Montlhéry to-day—which has deprived me of some of my audience—he noted, I say, that young people at such automobile track meets, etc., during the course of the emotion of excitement, which they feel, have a rise in their blood-sugar, which may even produce glycosuria. And this *emotive glycosuria* is simultaneously associated with alterations in the blood-adrenalin level.

There has been much discussion as to the existence of the *physiological adrenalinæmia*, that is to say the presence of certain amounts of adrenalin in normal blood, and the variations in this level. M. Gley, because he was unable to confirm the experimental observations of Tournade and Chabrol, would not admit the existence of variations in the level. But they produced further experimental evidence. They transfused blood from one dog to another, which of course eliminated any question of nervous effect, and having produced a hyperadrenalæmia in the donor, by stimulation of the peripheral end of the splanchnic, they noted, in the recipient dog, a vaso-motor reaction, characterized by hypertension and vaso-constriction. As a consequence, the stimulation of the great splanchnic causing an increase of adrenalin secretion, you can deter-mine the sympathetic reactions in the transfused dog.

This demonstrates that stimulation of the splanchnic produces hyperadrenalinæmia.

You are aware of the very close connections which exist between hyperadrenalinæmia and rise in blood sugar. There is a parallelism and Marañon has shown that emotion produces an increase in adrenalin through the splanchnics.

There does not seem to me to be any question about this, and why ? Why does an emotion-shock produce an increase in adrenalin ? Why does an emotion-shock particularly affect the adrenal, more than other endocrine glands ? Because there is a special arrangement of the sympathetic. The neurones of the great splanchnic have no synapses at the level of the chain ganglia ; they extend directly from the tractus intermedio-lateralis to the adrenal. This is a remarkable arrangement, which makes the great splanchnic an organized sympathetic system intermediate between the vagus system and the other federated sympathetic systems, which latter thus correspond to a somewhat loosely federated republic, whereas on the contrary the splanchnic system represents a government much more strongly organized and more in touch with the head.

Is this all ? No. It is not only a question of manifestations connected with nervous changes. There is more to it than that : the emotion-shock produces changes in surface tension and colloidal changes in the body fluids. Emotion-shocks, like all the shocks which are studied to-day in pathology, produce modifications in the blood-stream, from the point of view of its refractometric index, its viscosity, its colloidal state, and its ionic dissociation. In short, there actually does occur a *psychoclastic shock*, and, as M. Joltrain pointed out, during the war, in emotive cases there were not only nervous manifestations, but also humoral modifications, and that the old popular phrase : " My blood curdled " corresponds to a reality. You are familiar with the colloidoclastic formula of M. Widal with his modifications of the refractometric index, diminution in leucocytes, lowered pressure, variations in surface tension, viscosity, carbonic acid content, ionization, and naturally, changes in hydrogen-ion concentration, to which I shall return presently. You appreciate the appropriateness of the expression which I used, a long time ago, when I succeeded Prof. Dupré at the St. Anne Hospital, that alongside the nervous physiological psychiatry there is a *colloidal psychiatry*, and it is to this that one must turn to appreciate many manifestations, both normal and pathological.

But I am digressing. From this you see the observations to be made in studying the emotive, not in a unipolar way, but in their psychic manifestations of varying expression, and also in their somatic concomitants. Now that we appreciate what emotion is in the emotive, let us consider emotivity.

Emotivity is that *variation of the individual reaction co-efficient which is characterized by the intensity, the facility, and the frequency of emotion-shocks.* First, then, a description of emotivity before passing on to the study of its elements.

The description will be brief : one must, however, make the distinction between normal and morbid emotivity. *Normal emotivity* varies with age. *Infantile emotivity* contains, on the one hand, the predominance of the instincts, and on the other, the predominance of the vago-sympathetic reactions, type 3 (fig. vi). *Juvenile emotivity* is, on the whole, of the same order as infantile emotivity, with the appearance of the disturbing factor of the awakening of the sexual instinct with its variations in the secretions, which are very important in the male, and still more so in the female.

This brings me to *feminine emotivity*, whose existence as a separate entity is beyond all doubt. It is based—I say it somewhat unwillingly—perhaps on the predominance of the instincts, due to the fact of a less perfect development of the inter-neurone connections in the grey matter, and certainly to an increase in vago-sympathetic excitability, due chiefly to the ovarian and thyroid hormones.

Lastly, *senile emotivity* does not depend on an increase in secretions, but on a deficiency of the higher synthetic functions. This brings us to *morbid emotivity*, and here a distinction must be made depending on whether one is content with a superficial or surface study, or whether one makes a study in depth.

The *superficial clinical study* has been well made by Ernest Dupré, in his description of the *emotive constitution,*

which corresponds to a condition which one meets frequently, and which, from the pathological point of view,
constitutes a group which one can bring together under
the title of *emotive psychoneurosis*, a condition complicated
by anxiety manifestations of a paroxysmal nature, but
which are still contiguous.

If, instead of this, one makes a *clinical study in depth*,
one begins to see that these emotive people are extremely
diverse in their mechanisms, and that one must distinguish the reactions of the *psychic zone*—in which there
are variable insufficiencies in the personality under study;
—the manifestations of the *nervous zone*—with its variations in relation tone, and more important still with its
diffusions of sympathetic changes; the disturbances in
the *endocrine zone*—characterized often, from the morphological point of view, by persistence of an infantile
state (infantilism), often associated with hyperthyroidism
and, further, from the humoral aspect, a facility of occurrence of colloidoclastic shocks and lability of pH, that
is to say, of hydrogen-ion concentration, which varies
in such people with great facility; and in the *visceral zone*
by the frequency of such mechanical changes as ptosis,
for example, and such changes as are connected with
previous illnesses. And, lastly, if one studies the *morbific
kernel*, one becomes aware of a constitutional morbidity,
which expresses either intoxications—external such as
alcoholism, or internal as hyperthyroidism—or, traumata,
single trauma, such as railway accidents which produce a
morbid emotivity of several months or years' duration
after the accident, or successive traumata resulting in a
chronic state of emotivity, as was of frequent occurrence
during the war, where leaders of outstanding bravery
ended in a state in which the pop of a champagne cork
would upset them. In such cases there is an *acquired
morbid fear*, which has been studied by M. Broussaud in
his thesis on the subject, in which he shows its very important rôle, for it is not only of psychogenic origin, but
can be well explained by the changes in the internal

secretions caused by the emotion and by the ease with which adrenal disturbances occur, under the influence of emotive shocks, bringing in their train hyperadrenalinæmia.

You see the importance of this morbid emotivity, and if, instead of taking the standpoint of clinical study in depth, we take the *ætiological* point of view, we will distinguish an *arteriosclerotic* emotivity, an *alcoholic* emotivity, a *periodic* emotivity associated with *thyroid* disturbances, and a *traumatic* emotivity such as seen in war cases.

I come now to the *pathogenesis*, in order to see how one may group the different elements, which play a part in emotivity, for classification purposes.

First, we see that there is a possibility of an element of deficiency of the higher synthetic functions, and, second, endocrine changes typified by hyperthyroidism.

Let us review these elements. From the psychological point of view there appears a predominance of certain tendencies which in a way are more on the surface of consciousness than usual, due to a diminution or loss of activity of the higher synthetic functions. Then, there is a possibility of the repression of certain tendencies with secondary visceral disturbances. All these repression troubles are particularly studied by the Freudian School. It is here that one could come back to the definition, which I gave you a moment ago, of the emotions, that they are the " misfires of instinct."

Next come the sympathetic elements. These are orthosympathetic elements, with vaso-motor ataxy, vagal elements, allied to continued or paroxysmal anxiety, or endocrine elements, chiefly dominated by increased function of the thyroid and adrenals and disturbances in ovarian function.

The *emotivity of the menopause* has given us the classical mother-in-law type of comedy. This emotivity, related to insufficiency of the ovarian hormone, results in an overactivity of the thyroid. There is also an emotivity related to dysfunction of the ovary. Cases exist where the tendencies do not find relief, and where the endocrinologist may sometimes have recourse to substitutes (ersatz) ; certain products are of service in thus producing appeasement of special psycho-visceral agitations, when such cannot find better.

Next come the humoral manifestations, consisting chiefly in hyperadrenalinæmia, variations in blood-sugar, colloidoclastic shock, and variations in the hydrogen-ion concentration.

The variations in hydrogen-ion concentration are characterized by lability, that is to say, the very great field of the variations, and this is of service in distinguishing between hyperemotivity and anxiety. In the presence of a somatogenic anxiety reaction there is always an increase in the pH, which is usually over 7. In such cases, then, there is the urinary expression of a profound alkalosis, on which was based my statement that there existed an *alkaline anxiety neurosis*. But many emotives have variations only at certain hours or on certain days. Thus in several post-traumatic emotives, which I have observed, there were pH variations of from 4 up to 7½.

Now with regard to the modifications in unstripedmuscle fibre. In the emotive plain muscle is very often excited, with the occurrence of hair changes, rapid peristalsis causing diarrhœa. and violent vaso-motor and sweat reactions. Why is plain muscle fibre excited ? Is it only because it is under the influence of certain sympathetic fields ? By no means, for we observe plain-muscle-motor reactions in the vagal just as well as in the ortho-sympathetic field. One must look further afield for the reason. And one finds something remarkable. M. and Mme. Lapicque have observed changes in the faculty of *imbibition* of the muscle fibres. This *imbibition facility has a relationship to the chronaxy*. Let me recall to you that the chronaxy is limited by the rheobase. The *rheobase* is the quantity of electricity, measured in galvanic current, which is necessary to produce, for as long as one wishes, a contraction. It is the smallest current that will give a liminal contraction, that will pass the contraction threshold. Consequently it is the minimal amount of constant current, passing for as long as one wishes, to determine the liminal contraction threshold. You double the rheobase, that is to say you take twice that current, and with it you calculate the minimum time this constant current has to run to produce a threshold contraction. Thus you obtain the *chronaxy*, which thus is *the minimum time a constant current has to pass, the strength of which is twice the rheobase, to obtain the threshold contraction.*

This being established, you remeasure the chronaxy in relationship to variations of imbibition, and what do you find ? *The greater the qualities of imbibition are the proportionately shorter is the chronaxy.* On the other hand, you find that *imbibition is greater the higher the temperature*, and from that, you cannot avoid immediately establishing a relationship between what I said yesterday to my students, about the lengthening of the chronaxy, the slowness of the Erb reaction-like contraction, in people subjected to very prolonged immersion or cold, and showing the physiopathic syndromes of Babinski. Thus you see how things link themselves up.

Furthermore, what else do you observe ? You see this, that if we perfuse smooth-muscle fibres with Ringer's fluid, in which we vary either the calcium-ions, or the potassium-ions, there is a diminution of response with the calcium-ions, and an augmentation with the potassium-ions. Now, we know that the same is true for the chronaxy, and as a result we can see a very close parallelism, and hence we come to outline the idea of a *physical theory of emotivity*, a physical theory based on the qualities of imbibition of plain muscle, thus allowing the production of variations in the chronaxy, and playing a considerable rôle in the manifestations of *emotive behaviour* of individuals.

Obviously, this does not explain everything, but we

know that in the young, the chronaxy is short, and that there is facility of imbibition ; consequently, one cannot avoid noticing that there are in this some very interesting facts, which help us to avoid too narrow divisions of the psychic, neurological, and even endocrine fields, and instead of spreading ourselves in the field of surface manifestations, to penetrate the domain of that *psycho-physico-chemical life,* which is coming to occupy the first place in the biological explanations for which we are searching.

Thus, you see where our observations are leading. We already have a certain number of words descriptive of these clinical types which differ according to the point of view. The psychologists speak of the *hyper-emotive* with the Freudian anxiety neuroses. The sympathologists speak of the *vaso-motor sympathetic* type. The endocrinologists speak of *hyperthyroidism.* The physiologists, with leanings towards physical views, speak of hypermotivity of plain muscle. Lastly, others, clinicians with physical view-points, speak of the *colloidoclastic* diathesis.

All these syndromes are very closely similar. They somewhat resemble those soldiers who fought with each other, because their crown-pieces were not of the same colour but, when they had turned the coins over, they perceived that some were coloured red on the obverse, while others were blue on the reverse, and that it was only necessary to turn them to have them all similar. Here, the same is true. Nevertheless, I do not want to be a " simplist." I do not wish to say that all these types are identical ; hyperemotivity, vasomotor sympathetic type, hyperthyroidism and hypermotivity of plain muscle, and colloidoclastic diathesis. I say, simply, that they are very close, although in all probability their margins would not exactly coincide, if one were to superimpose them on each other in order to establish their contours, in the manner of Galton's method. Nevertheless, I believe that this has a certain importance, and at least you see how various people consider emotivity and the factors which play a part in its production, from which follow, naturally, practical and theoretical conclusions.

The *practical conclusions*, with reference to treatment, which should be thorough, have regard to the individual in the entirety of his situation ; educative treatment of the character, self-control, hydrotherapy. Further, such treatment as will tend to reduce repression to the minimum, helping the patient to sublimate the instinctive emotions, and perhaps also making constructive use of the dreams ; for the dream has a cathartic function, and the frequent dreamer may by this means, during the night, rid himself of many ideas and emotions, and so, sometimes, may save himself from committing follies during the day.

Next I want to emphasize the importance of treatment directed towards the sympathetic, by means of certain sedative drugs, the most undoubtedly valuable of which is opium in small doses ; laudanum in doses of 15 to 20 minims is sometimes a remarkable brake on certain emotivities, and I know patients who owe to it such a threshold of emotivity as enables them to have a normal life.

On the glandular side, I would mention atropine or hæmato-ethyroidine, to diminish thyroid hyperexcitability and, finally, from the point of view of smooth muscle function, to strengthen the organismal order of control I suggest the exhibition of calcium-ions, which is certainly a marvellous nerve tonic which tones up the controlling functions.

Also from the practical point of view, alongside the therapeutic, there is the question of the *medico-legal deduction.* Formerly, using Charcot's classification of such cases, when there was noted an absence of physical signs of involvement of the nervous system, one said " This is a case of hysteria," and there was a tendency to incline to the view that the indemnity was reduced to zero. It was to the credit of the old medico-legal experts that they called attention to the fact that following railway accidents, producing in the patient serious disturbance,

D

there was often a persistence of a tachycardia, and neurasthenia with tachycardia was looked on as in a different category.   To-day we explain the condition fully as being associated with disturbances of the thyroid and adrenals ; consequently, alongside the *organo-genetic* manifestations, are the *physio-genetic* manifestations which ought to be distinguished from modifications purely *psycho-genetic*, and which ought to be followed, not only by a diminution in working capacity, but also by a correlative compensation.

And lastly, the *theoretical conclusion :* it is that you see the importance of these questions, which are, in a fashion, the intersection of a series of avenues, which lead to important general ideas.

It is always a pleasure to play with general ideas in the gardens of Academos.   And I believe that you might retain of this lecture, which I feel has been much too long —nevertheless I thank you for your remarkable attention —you might remember, in a way as its essential thought, that *emotivity* might be called the *flames of the heart*, but that *affectivity without emotivity* is still better, and that one might express this state comparatively as the smokeless *ignis ardens*.

III

THE CONCENTRIC METHOD IN THE DIAGNOSIS
OF PSYCHONEUROTICS

*" The Burgraves had three armours : the first built
of courage was their heart ; the second of steel, clothed
them ; the third of granite, their fort."*

VICTOR HUGO.

I WISH to address you to-day on the Concentric Method
of diagnosis of people suffering from psychoneuroses.
Let me recall to you that, the other day, I divided the
psychoneuroses into four varieties, taking as my basis
simply, if one may call it so, the *surface diagnosis*. This
classification gave : Hysteria, with suggestibility and
delusion in predominance ; Neurasthenia, with depression
predominating ; Psychasthenia, with anxious doubt predominating ; and Emotive Psychoneurosis characterized
by emotion and the visceral disturbances which accompany it.

In connection with the four patients representative of
these four types, whom I showed you, I told you that in
going into the matter more deeply, each of them could be
shown to be involved in processes of much greater complexity, in which there was constantly to be noted a
visceral element. And in proof of this I ended my lecture
in demonstrating to you a woman whose condition was a
synthesis of these four types, in which one found, as components, elements of hysteria, neurasthenia, psychasthenia, as well as emotive psychoneurosis.

All of which shows the necessity in every case of
psychoneurosis to apply, what I call the " Diagnosis in

Depth " and not merely to be content with a superficial diagnosis.

In order to grasp the significance of this diagnosis in depth, I must first recall to your minds what is the classical rule in the establishment of any diagnosis. I have already given this but its importance will justify the stress of repetition.

Diagnosis is essentially the correlation of each individual clinical case with the generalities of descriptive pathology. Take as an example : a woman with shortness of breath, cyanosis of the lips, œdema of the lower limbs, increase in heart and liver dullness, scanty urine, and a rapid small pulse. One diagnoses the syndrome : in this case it is a disturbance of cardiac function expressing itself in defective cardiac systole. On auscultation of the organ a systolic murmur is found at the apex, conducted to the axilla, in short the condition is Mitral Insufficiency. Thus the *affection* is diagnosed, or in other words the site of the morbid process is localized.

But on questioning the patient one learns that she has had Acute Articular Rheumatism, and so one reasonably concludes that the *cause* of her trouble is an acute infection. So that when one thinks as a clinician one proceeds from the individual to the general descriptions, using the *inductive method*, and from the syndrome; in actuality an expression of disturbed functions, one passes to the affection, which is the localization of the morbid site in an organ, and thence one passes to the disease or causal agent, which may be, for example, an intoxication, infection, cancer or vitamine deficiency.

In the above case then the diagnosis should run : Heart failure from mitral incompetence of rheumatic origin.

If, however, one thinks as a pathologist, one will use the *deductive method* and pass successively from disease to affection and thence to syndrome, realizing how the disease is produced by noting its effect on the viscera it singles out, and how these latter in turn give rise to the syndrome.

However, in Psychiatry, there is not only a syndrome-diagnosis to be made but also a *clinical-picture-diagnosis* which derives from the social reactions of the patient. This is because the brain is not an organ such as other organs are, for it has a special function in interpsychological relationships, and thus, in psychiatry, one would describe an individual, showing ideas of grandeur or persecution with intellectual deficiency, as demented, when compared with another suffering say from diffuse meningo-encephalitis, or general paralysis of luetic origin.

But this is not all. If one poleaxes an individual he falls down unconscious, whatever his individuality may be, for the violence is intense enough to eliminate any reactions due to personality, which of course would vary in different individuals. On the other hand, proportionately as the traumatic cause is diminished the individual reactions will occupy a larger field of the clinical picture, to the extent that the diagnosis will not be complete unless it finally states : *clinical picture-type* with *syndrome, affection, disease, in a person* possessing such and such a *constitution*, such and such a *temperament*, and such and such a *character*, the constitution being the morphological expression, the temperament the physiological expression, and the character the psychological expression of the individual reactional coefficient. Only when one has gone right through under these seven heads can one make a complete clinical diagnosis.

But although this may be easy in many cases, yet very often it is impossible, owing to the intricacy of symptoms in people who are very nervous, to connect the syndrome with disturbance of functions and to establish its relationship with an affection. The necessity therefore arises for a method by which one prudently classifies all the symptoms referable to certain zones. I have been led to adopt this method from studying the question of industrial accidents, and in a lecture in 1919 on the nervous and psychic reactions in such cases, I showed that in a case of industrial accident one had first to apply the method of Babinski : ascertain whether or not physical signs were present of an organic nervous system lesion affection. This then is the first kernel, the *central organic lesion kernel.*

In other words one had to ascertain if the behaviour of the patient was consistent with an organic process, or more allied to some particular interest, to a selfish interest. In short, the fact that had struck all observers, since the law of 1898, on industrial accidents, is that, for the same accident, whatever it may be, there is a considerable difference in the length of time necessary for recovery, according to whether the patient can benefit in some way from his accident or not. Brissaud made this important statement and it shows that there are certain mental reactions that occur in patients suffering from accidents, and that around this central organic lesion kernel, with functional physical signs, there is an atmosphere rendered more or less hazy by the doubtful connection with reactions occurring in the intelligence and mind of the individual intent on making the best of the situation.

But, you say, it is surely unnecessary to recapitulate all this theory simply to restate what was being said in the time of Charcot when they already spoke of the association of hysterical elements in organic manifestations.

To do so, however, is most useful for between this organic kernel and this sphere of " behaviour manifestations," to use the term of Lacassagne, there lies another zone—a zone that Vibert had noted. For it had been observed that, in individuals suffering from traumatic psychoneurosis, whether classifiable as hysteria or traumatic neurasthenia, there were some who exhibited a tachycardia that nothing could quieten ; that there was also a degree of emotivity surpassing considerably that which the individual could determine himself and which took a very long time indeed to subside ; and finally the prognosis appeared to differ according to whether the case showed this abnormal tachycardia or not.

Cannon's animal experiments in which he determined

the particular psychic manifestations which follow adrenalin injection, and in the converse sense the observations made by certain writers on the discharge of adrenalin in emotional states, have demonstrated that this observation of Vibert's was justified, and that there existed a functional process, which was by no means *psychogenetic*, that is to say it had no connection with phenomena associated either with the intelligence, a wish, or an interest, but that on the contrary it was *physiogenetic*,

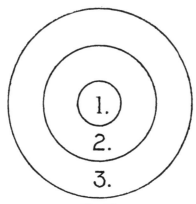

Fig. II

CONCENTRIC SCHEMA OF INDUSTRIAL ACCIDENT CASE
1. Central organic-lesional kernel.
2. Physiogenetic zone.
3. Behaviour manifestations.

that is to say, arising from disturbance of the organism itself.

This physiogenetic sphere is very important in that it is closely bound up to sympathetic and endocrine symptomatology. It is independent of organo-lesional changes as it is of psychic disturbances, but it is intimately related to *functional organic disturbances*. Thus one may call it a *sphere of dynamic disturbances*, which led me to state that, in industrial accidents, the individual reacts with the whole of his being, with his body (organic lesion), with his heart (dynamic organic disturbance), and with his mind (psychogenetic disturbance).

It is this that has led me to the concentric method in the diagnosis of the psychoneurotics, in which it is necessary to distinguish five zones.   First there is the *peripheral psychic atmosphere*, then beneath this the *nervous zone*, thirdly the *endocrine zone*, then the *visceral zone*, and lastly and innermost the *central morbific kernel*.

In order to help you to understand the usefulness of this division I should like to present for your consideration the case of Mlle. Germaine, whom, if you have no objection, we shall call Sylvie, for in certain ways she resembles this heroine of Gérard de Nerval.   She has some of her qualities and, like the real Sylvie, she was a native of that Ile de France whose soft skies seemed to cast their glow on her soul and found their reflection in the delicacy of her sentiments.

She is a young patient, frail and somewhat pallid, whose cheek flushes with the lightest emotion that brushes her heart ; she talks quite readily.   This is her history.   She is a pianoforte teacher twenty-four years old.   Her trouble began in 1919 and she describes it :   " While out shopping I felt a growing malaise that got worse the more I walked ; till, arriving at my destination, this feeling was dreadful, terrifying.   People did not know what on earth to do for me—they thought I was going to die.   In a few minutes I was seized with a trembling and I had the feeling that everything around me was ' queer.'   They found it very hard to get me back to my normal state.

" Later these attacks returned and were terrible and from then on it became impossible for me to go out.   As soon as I arrived at the end of my street I was forced to return home ; on several occasions friends forced me to go on but only with dreadful results.   Occasionally when I had turned back the attack eased but did not disappear.   There were some streets I did not dare enter.   It became absolutely impossible for me to remain at home alone ; the moment I was left my hands became ice-cold, my face flushed, and I don't know what happened to me, but it was as if I were delirious.   I would have gone in anywhere or I would have taken anybody into our house. My heart beat terribly. The chief sensation of it all was and still is that I was going to die."

This description is interesting, because it can be schematized by an outside crisis, with phobia, on the one hand, while, on the other hand, there are some very clean-cut manifestations—that sensation that "everything around me has become changed," which has been so fully studied by Pierre Janet, and which can be classified under what he has termed *Psycholepsy*, which is a state associated with a diminution in the psychological tension.

But to continue the history of this case :

" Later on these attacks appeared not only while I was out but also in the house, and to such an extent that going out at all became almost impossible." (This is agoraphobia.) " Scarcely had I gone a few yards when I was forced to return."

At this time it was impossible for Sylvie to remain at home alone ; she had disorderly heart action, vaso-motor disturbances, and to inhibit these manifestations it was merely necessary for her to have someone with her. In short, this shows clearly the psychogenetic character of these troubles. The same phenomena were produced when someone came to visit her. She could not endure anyone for more than a few minutes ; she was forced to leave the room, for otherwise " she did not know what would have happened to her."

In 1920, 1921, 1922, 1923, this condition continued with some slight improvement. We find in this case a cyclic tendency in the manifestations: at certain times she is more depressed than at others.

On the 19th August, 1924, her father, who was an alcoholic, died ; all her symptoms became worse but at the same time quite changed their character; her subjective feelings became infinitely varied, with only a slight general resemblance between them, and very difficult and in fact sometimes quite impossible to describe.

This difficulty of description is indeed the rule in these manifestations, in which there is an important sympathetic element.

To a certain extent these troubles are connected with the menstrual functions. Sylvie has, before her period, and particularly fifteen days before, a slight discharge accompanied by a rise of temperature—to 38 deg. C. Then some ten days before the period, that is some five days after the temperature and discharge, she has an attack of gastric discomfort accompanied by redness and pain in the epigastrium; thereafter there are several days of remission in which she is well enough, the menstrual flow begins and the temperature falls to normal.

After the period there are some days of moderate well-being, but about fifteen days after the period the nervous attacks reappear.

Since the middle of 1925 there has been a reappearance of the nervous attacks, and we enter into the second period, one of *depression*, in which attacks come on, to use the hallowed phrase, on the slightest provocation : crying spells and internal spasms end in a nervous attack.

There is, then, a picture which corresponds to the *attack of hysteria*. The patient sometimes has the impression that the attack is not going off well ; the nerves are tense and there is confusion, and there is that particular feeling of not being as before. During the whole attack the anxiety is extreme and there is the feeling of approaching dissolution. Then the attack ends, order is restored, and there appears a feeling of well-being, an impression of being relieved ; it was this feeling that gave rise to the expression, used by sufferers from similar attacks in the Middle Ages, of the devil having gone out of them and that they were delivered.

Sometimes, in the present case, instead of the attack terminating there would appear a loss of nervous equilibrium that would last some two weeks, during which the most curious and acutely uncomfortable manifestations appeared, with difficulty in digestion, and discomfort localized in the left side between the heart and the stomach. There is extreme weakness, then suddenly the attack subsides.

Since August, 1926, the time when Sylvie first consulted us, she has still from time to time attacks of what she calls *internal congestion*, with pain in the back, stomach, intestine, and ovary, attacks that are accompanied by palpitations and vaso-motor disturbances ; veins become distended and the feet are cold. Such are symptoms that one is very familiar with in people suffering from colitic affections and who are air-swallowers. This manifestation is due to vago-sympathetic reactions caused by stimulation from the inflamed colon.

The menstrual function has become very irregular, the discharge being scanty in amount ; coincidentally, there is extreme lassitude and a general revulsion from most things ; this is the strain of *melancholia* which has resulted from the period of depression, which is a common experience of this patient. A restful night is a rare occurrence ; she often wakes in the middle of the night bathed in sweat, and with a feeling of fearful malaise—an example of these sudden awakenings at two in the morning that patients suffering from gastro-intestinal pathologies know so well—every nerve from head to heels seems on the stretch, with the feeling of cramp between heart and stomach ; motor reactions occur which penetrate the level of consciousness and give rise to those cenæsthetic feelings that, originating in gaseous distension of the stomach and colon, are registered as empty feeling in the head and heart, anxiety, a wish to die, and a feeling that one cannot endure a moment more.

Ultimately the patient begins to realize that these symptoms have, up to a certain point, a relationship to food, the condition being generally worst before and after meals and towards six in the evening. Also, an important point, the condition is aggravated in the erect posture. Why ? Because Sylvie has a well-marked visceroptosis which drags on her solar plexus, and which causes disturbance through that plexus in a perfectly natural way. At least there would seem to be, she says, "an alternate swinging in her condition from troubles localized to certain organs to the nervous part of her trouble, characterized by attacks of headache and nerves, and the formation of a ball on her stomach."

This of course is very interesting, because it is indeed from varying degrees of solar plexus reaction that effects will predominate either on the sensory-motor system or on the vago-sympathetic ; and it is such reactions that have played a rôle in the theory of *metastases* which Broussais held.

" In spite of all her troubles this patient had a very good appetite," which fact allows one to differentiate between the dyspepsias of diseases of the nervous system, and the digestive troubles that owe their occurrence to changes in the digestive tube.

Nevertheless, in spite of this good appetite, there has been a loss of eight kilos in this patient ; and this loss of weight in presence of good appetite is one of the criteria of the greatest importance in psychic depression : loss of weight accompanied by lassitude and rapid fatiguability.

This patient was seen in the out-patient department, when one was struck by the loss of weight and her special *morphology* ; other outstanding points were lack of development of the breasts ; hairy overgrowths on the mammary areolæ and in the intermammary space, as well as a scoliosis, indicating an important disturbance of endocrine function.

With regard to evidence of *sympathetic* function deficiency, her systolic blood pressure is low—12—with a diastolic of 8.[1] In the recumbent position the pulse was 108, while upright it was 128.

There are evidences of certain vaso-motor disturbances ;

[1] These pressures are taken with the Pachon Oscillometer which is graduated in centimetres. Multiplication by ten will give the pressure in mm. Hg.—Trans.

the palms of the hands are moist, and the feet are cold. The *solar plexus reflex* showed a marked diminution in the oscillations from 4 to 2. On the other hand the *oculo-cardiac reflex* gave a figure somewhat on the high side, as on ocular compression, the pulse fell from 80 to 56 : one may therefore conclude that there is hyperexcitability of the vago-sympathetic.

Clinical examination of the gastro-intestinal tract reveals stomach " splashing " on movement, constipation, gaseous distension of the colon and the presence of Level's sign—diminution of pain at the level of the solar plexus when the intestines are supported in an upward direction by the examiner.

Radioscopic examination, carried out by my pupil, M. Arbeit, in every way confirms this direct clinical examination. The stomach is large and extends as far downwards as four finger-breadths beneath the line joining the iliac crests, while in the prone position its position is some 5 or 6 cms. higher. There is no deformity of the gastric curvatures, the liver is normal, and there is no point of localized pain in the stomach. Gastric movements are poor, pylorospasm is present, and attrition of its contents is delayed by its slow and difficult emptying. In the fasting state there is stasis of the contents.

The duodenum shows no morphological abnormality, and spasmodic contraction is absent except for a slight degree in the third portion, without pain, however. There is stasis in the small bowel. We have in short the classical picture of *gaseous distension of the colon*.

The large intestine, which occupies only a somewhat low position in the prone posture, shows well marked ptosis when the patient is upright, in which position the two colic flexures are beneath the level of the iliac crests, and the reduction of this ptosis, which is possible in decubitus, is very difficult, in fact impossible, when she is in the erect posture. The descending colon is normal and appears to empty itself normally. On the other hand a certain degree of stasis can be noted in the ascending colon with distension of the cæcum.

This latter point is noteworthy for in the consideration of *colic stasis* it is of extreme importance to note whether the condition affects the ascending or descending part, for while stasis in the *latter* does not produce any very marked nervous reactions, stasis of the *cæcum and ascending part* has a very profound influence not only on the nervous system but also on the general nutrition of the patient.

The cæco-appendicular region is normal, but there is evidence of some slight adhesion of the hepatic flexure of the colon to the gall-bladder.

In addition, a most important observation, the right third of the transverse colon shows irregularities of contour, which would seem to indicate the presence of *pericolitis*. You recall, of course, from M. Carnot's remarkable work, the great importance of pericolitis in abdominal symptomatology; this is a point that is well worth bringing out, and for further details on this subject I refer you to the book this author has recently published with M. Blamoutier.

These periviscerites, then, play a very important rôle in sympathetic pathology. Even the palpation of this segment of bowel is painful and produces protective contraction of the abdominal wall, and visible spasm of the transverse colon, which although extremely ptosed does not appear to have any adhesions in its middle third.

The descending colon shows spasm, in its iliac portion, and finally the sigmoid is normal.

You now see the point of this examination of the digestive tube, which indeed is deservedly connected with the observations of sympathetic pathology we have made.

Further it has to be noted that the gall-bladder is not only enlarged in size but is opaque to the rays.

Examination of the chest shows a slight diffuse shadow at the left apex, not cleared up on coughing; a haziness at the right apex clears considerably better; lastly, there is one patch which shows small areas of calcification in its outer part ; it is here that we come upon the " morbid kernel " in this patient's case.

If we pass this case history in review, using our schema of five zones, we can say that :

In the *psychic zone* we note an emotive psychoneurosis with attacks of anxiety, in which is also distinguishable elements of hysteria, phobia, visceral perturbations and depression. Using our method of diagnosis, we note the presence of the hysterical, neurasthenic, psychasthenic, and psycho-emotive elements with attacks of anxiety in a woman suffering from *overaction of the sympathetic* nervous system, that is with both vagotonia and ortho-sympathicotonia.

In the *endocrine zone* she shows herself to be dysfunctional, somewhat gynandroid in type (indicated by under-development of the breasts and hairy overgrowth in the areolar and intermammary regions) with slight ovarian disturbances.

In the *visceral zone* there is visceroptosis with gaseous distension of the colon and biliary lithiasis.

The "*morbid kernel*" is pulmonary tuberculosis and scoliosis in a hereditary alcoholic.

I could stress the other uses of this method by giving you other case histories, but I think it preferable to use all we have noted in this typical case as a basis for a synthetic development of the method ; and for this we must now return to the different zones we have already studied, to see how we must handle our analysis in each.

1. PSYCHIC ZONE.—The psychic zone is composed of two aspects :

(*a*) An *external aspect* with a bearing on social and interpsychological relationships.

(*b*) An *internal aspect*.

The external aspect is very often complicated by a series of manifestations due to the *familial* or *professional inter-psychology*, to such an extent that when one first sees the patient, it is often extremely difficult to realize the depth to which the troubles extend. The position of a psycho-neurotic on being institutionalized is very similar to that of a tuberculous patient on admission to a sanatorium. Guinard, de Desmarets, and de Sabourin pointed out that,

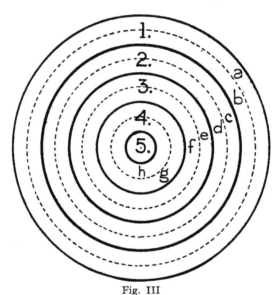

Fig. III

DIAGRAM OF THE FIVE ZONES

1. Psychic Zone.
   (a) Exterior Aspect, interpsychological.
   (b) Interior Aspect, deep.
2. Nervous Zone.
   (c) Aspect of Neurological Relationship.
   (d) Sympathetic Aspect.
3. Endocrine Zone.
   (e) Humoral Aspect.
   (f) Morphological Aspect.
4. Visceral Zone.
   (g) Physiological Aspect.
   (h) Anatomo-Pathological Aspect.
5. Morbific Kernel.

before one could be able to form an opinion of the condition of a case of pulmonary tuberculosis and make a prognosis, it was necessary for the patient to pass a few days in the institution to give him time to " rid himself " of the signs caused by some superadded bronchitis

Similarly, the psychoneurotic should be allowed, during the first week or two of his stay in the institution, to " rid himself " of his familial and professional interpsychological reactions, and during this period one notes the modifications that occur in his conduct and work, and one studies with the greatest care his behaviour in his daily actions.

We are indebted to Freud for drawing attention to " *slips*," *lapsus* of the tongue and in conduct, which illuminate the depths of the psychological being, and one is further able to penetrate this *internal aspect* of the psychology by using the method of *association words*, which can be an important factor in the analysis of the sub-conscious, and the various interesting procedures which enable one to study dream-states and reveries, keeping in mind Renan's saying " that one must not put too high a value on one who has not the habit, from time to time, of praying."

2. NERVOUS ZONE.—Here also two aspects come up for consideration : the *aspect of neurological relationship*, and the *sympathetic aspect*.

(*a*) In the *aspect of neurological relationship*, one must look for criteria characterized by the presence or absence of physical signs of organic lesional affection of the nervous system.

(*b*) In the *sympathetic aspect*, one ascertains if the sympathetic manifestations are of a lesional or dynamic order.

3. ENDOCRINE ZONE.—Here, again, there are two aspects to be viewed : a *humoral aspect* and a *morphological aspect*.

(*a*) *Humoral aspect*.—The internal secretions by their hormones, hormazones and chalones, that is secretions which stimulate or inhibit other glands, or control the growth of the individual, modify the humoral composition. This latter must consequently be studied by all physical, chemical, and other procedures possible, especially stressing the study of pH, that is hydrogen-ion concentration both in blood and urine.

E

(b) *Morphological aspect.*—This morphological aspect is one of the characteristic features of endocrine disturbances. And here the important law of the botanist de Vries tends to displace the Darwinian idea, which former states that morphological modifications, whose appearance is noted in the evolution of beings, are above all a function of modifications of their physico-chemical constitution. Morphology, then, being merely an expression of endocrine physico-chemical equilibrium, it is therefore in this aspect that we shall be able to note the factors originating from constitution, temperament and character. And we see that the individual co-efficient of reaction becomes more important as the morbid cause is less in evidence.

4. VISCERAL ZONE.—Here again there are two aspects : the *physiological* and the *anatomo-pathological.*

(a) *Physiological aspect.*—In the case we have discussed (Sylvie) it is, gaseous distension of the colon, visceroptosis, and air swallowing.

(b) *Anatomo-pathological aspect.*—This is of great importance and must always be studied with care. In Sylvie's case there is found on the one hand pulmonary lesions, and on the other gall-bladder pathology. In a carefully considered study therefore it will be of importance to decide whether these conditions are merely co-incidental or whether they may have a pathogenic significance.

5. MORBIFIC KERNEL.—We now arrive at the morbific kernel, as we designate the diseases, which, in this particular case, are labelled pulmonary tuberculosis, as the acquired complaint, and hereditary alcoholism as the inherited disease.

Thus, we have concluded the complete analysis of our patient. What conclusions are we to draw from it ?

Conclusions.—Having made the above analysis, in which every feature has been relegated to its proper sphere, there only remains the need of establishing the ætiological order of the components. This order evidently demands, not only a critical, but one may well say, also an intuitive mind, for it is in this most of all that there is room for difference of opinion. The advantage of the Concentric Method, however, is that, whatever may be the secondary interpretation which the clinician may put on the concentric formulæ put before him, they will still remain valid, for in them we have an accumulation of documented facts methodically presented, of which each person, according to his viewpoint, will lay stress on this or that part.

Were our patient to consult an internist, she would certainly be considered as a case of gas distension of the bowel and visceroptosis with digestive trouble, while on consulting us, neurologists, we should certainly lay stress on the importance of the neurological and psychopathic symptoms.

There is, then, a contingent element in the order ; but no matter how one views the relationships in it, it is certain that the concentric method has one considerable advantage. It is that it is a synthetic method which illuminates the individual's componential factors. This permits, on the one hand, a treatment that will not be one-sided, which will take into account not only the mind or the nervous system, or the visceral, or the endocrine systems, or the organic lesions alone, but will allow of a synthetic treatment into which will concomitantly enter psychotherapy, hygiene, dietetics, physiotherapy, endocrine therapy, as well as Galenic pharmacy.

This combination of psychotherapy and endocrine therapy is by no means a new thing, for Galen gave a very clear description of it.

This concentric method permits of the institution of a therapy for each individual case, in place of a same-for-all therapy—which ought not to exist.

Now I hope I have shown you the whole advantage of this method. On the next occasion we shall study in detail each of these zones, and the relationships between consciousness and the unconscious.

IV

CONSCIOUSNESS AND THE UNCONSCIOUS SELF IN PSYCHONEUROTICS

A COURSE of lectures, covering years, would not exhaust this subject. Therefore I shall try to confine myself chiefly to the practical aspects of this question. After a general outline of the principal psychic manifestations we shall draw from these the methods of examination which seem to me to be the best. I shall then give you several examples of the application of these methods and we shall draw from the statement of the facts several inductions.

Every being, from the very fact that he is, tends to continue in his existence. That is one of the axioms of Spinoza in his " Ethics." It is certain that the tendency to persist is one of the primordial qualities of living beings, and if one studies the tendencies, one becomes aware that one can, in arranging them in their order of importance, establish as a series important divisions in psychophysiology. This is what has been done in recent years by Pierre Janet in his course of physiology at the College de France.

In the first place one can distinguish the *higher tendencies*, which find their expression in logic and ethics, which appear *a priori* to depend essentially on psychological activity, and have no relationship to the organism.

At the other extreme are the *lower tendencies* which, in the ordinary way, neurologists group with the functions of the nervous system and which are associations—more or less complex—of reflexes. The reflexes consist of a centripetal arc running to the nerve centre and a centrifugal arc going from the nerve centre to the periphery. When a second arc is in circuit with this reflex arc, it often happens that the stimulation acts on the motor neurone in a non-specific manner, that is to say, there is substitution ; the neurone responds to a peripheral stimulus, which has taken the place of the first habitual, classical stimulus ; this is what Pavlov has called a " conditioned reflex." This reflex plays a rôle of considerable importance in psychology, for it is the basis of the phenomena of habit, and habit is the memory of the organism.

All these lower tendencies, which are already extremely complex, can, nevertheless, be tied up with a more or less definite part of the organism, can be connected with viscera. But what interests us above all are the *inter-mediate tendencies*, that is intermediate between the higher tendencies, of the ethical and logical sphere, and the lower tendencies of the animal life.

These intermediate tendencies are characterized, on the one hand, by the fact that, from the point of view of their origin, they spring from the depths of the organism-from its cenesthesia, and on the other hand that, in their expression, they liberate themselves from the regional parts of the organism by a character of universality, in which they resemble the higher tendencies.

It is this domain of intermediate tendencies which is alone affected in the psychoneurotics.

But it is not enough to schematize the psychic life by the order of tendencies ; it has to be taken into account that, when one dreams, when one lets oneself drift on the tide of thought, a current-like condition is established in the mind, and this flow of images, impressions, emotions, memories, resembles in every way fluid currents. It was the great merit of William James that he opposed the atomic psychology of Taine, who did psychic stencilling, in reducing everything to distinct psychic facts. William James showed the opposite to be the case, that the psychic life was a perpetual stream, in which mingled superficial currents and deep currents more or less illuminated by consciousness and that there existed between consciousness and unconsciousness regions of shadow.

This discovery, which has surprised lay philosophers, long out of contact with theological studies, is a commonplace idea in religious writers. I do not need to remind you that, if St. Dominic invented the rosary, it was because he had the intuition of the different levels of the currents in the human soul, and because he knew that the best way of allowing the deep currents to group themselves, as it were, around a simple idea, is to occupy the superficial currents with an automatic activity such for example as the repetition of the Pater and the Ave. It is for this reason that I often call the chaplet " the stairs of prayer."

This existence of superficial and deep currents has impressed Bergson, who has borrowed much from the Mystics, and with good reason he has distinguished the fragmentary discursive current of the intelligence, cutting out in the superficial currents fragments of reality.

He has thus defined the intelligence as an instrument which seizes the moving moment that is always flowing by. The character of discursive intelligence is, indeed, to seize momentary impressions, in the superficial currents of the being.

This is useful practically, for it is thanks to it that the Greeks discovered reason. But it has the inconvenience of simply transferring into space manifestations whose modality is time ; hence the paradox of the Eleates, in the story of the hare and the tortoise, in that in dividing indefinitely the distance separating the hare from the tortoise, never, from the point of view of logic, must the hare catch up with the tortoise. This paradox shows that the rational method of the discursive intelligence can seize a part of the phenomena ; nevertheless, by reason of its schematism, it never succeeds in seizing the reality in the whole of its depth and is content to seize it in only one of its modalities in order to gain advantages from it in current life.

Apart from these superficial currents which solidify in a series of blocks, there are deep currents, currents which are not always, in a general way, in the depth. Certain of them, indeed, correspond in the soul to what are, in geology, those subterranean rivers, so fully studied by Martel, and which, at certain times, may reappear on the surface. They are not springs ; it is only the appearance in consciousness of a subconscious current. Now, if the individual is unaware of the deep current up to the moment when it breaks the surface of his consciousness, he has the impression that there is produced in him a psychological element, which is independent of himself, and since, in deep meditation, this instant bursts on him, it becomes : in the artist, inspiration and in the religious, passive contemplation. It is, one might say, the point of insertion of the human and the divine.

But this is not all. There are states, and particularly states of prayer—they may be æsthetic or religious—in which there occurs something like an eruption of the unconscious, which quickly passes across consciousness and enlightens the individual, as if he had received a vision from on high. It is this state which is known as *ecstasy*, in which from the fact of the intensity of concentration of the individual in some manner on an idea, there is a true eruption of the unconscious self through consciousness and beyond.

This ecstatic eruption includes psychic currents which are divisible into three segments.

Myers, who has made an extensive study of mediumship, compares the psyche of the individual to an iceberg, of which the greater part is under the surface of the waves, while the lesser part gleams iridescent in the sun. This latter corresponds to consciousness, while the part that is submerged corresponds to the subliminal self. One might even say that above the consciousness, especially in people who attain to ecstasy, there is a region that takes on again the character of the subliminal self, and which I shall call the *ultra-liminal* region, comparable to what is found in the spectrum where there are ultra-violet rays beyond the violet.

There are, then, three degrees : the *infra-conscious* region, corresponding to the infra-red ; the *conscious region*, and the *ultra-conscious* region.

This leads me to show you the importance of consciousness in this flow of psychic phenomena. Consciousness would appear to be born of the contingency of the direction of nervous influx. Once the reflex is determined, there is no consciousness of it. When the engrams establish themselves in the brain, in such a way that they direct the nervous influx, consciousness of it disappears. Under the influence of habit we lose consciousness of the things we do.

It is interesting to see that consciousness would appear to be born of the contingency of the paths followed by the nervous influx and that it is just this same contingency which is the reason used by human beings to mount to the conception of God. The demonstration of this fact, establishing these two conceptions of soul and God, shows that they are connected with two neighbouring manifestations. This consciousness must be distinguished according to its degree of diffusion, or its degree of concentration.

Consciousness, more or less diffuse, extends in the shadow region of William James as far as those regions which are not illuminated at all. But the interesting point is above all the study of concentrated consciousness, concentrated as is the light which passes through the Abbé condenser of a microscope.

When one concentrates one's consciousness on a point, by this very act a part of the psychic field is in a state of inaction. *Distraction* appears. This phenomenon of distraction has a particular importance and presents different signs, according to whether it is a question of voluntary concentration of consciousness on a point which one wishes to solve, or whether the distraction results from a pathological disturbance.

This, in passing, shows that, to designate a special

pathological character as schizoid is only a useful statement of psychiatry, but that this *schizoid character*—
character of a person who falls readily into distraction—
is only a state of exaggeration of what one must consider
as normal.

You are now aware of the distinction to establish between consciousness and the unconscious self, one corresponding to the *social aspect* and the other to the *intimate
aspect* of the *psychic zone.*

In connection with the *concentric method* in the diagnosis
of psychoneurotics, I told you that it was always necessary
to search the different zones, psychic, neurological, endocrine, visceral, and morbific, and that the psychic zone
was divided into two aspects : the peripheral or social
aspect, and the deep or internal aspect.   It has long been
known that these two aspects existed and one may designate them in the manner I have indicated, showing you,
however, that there are varying degrees of delimitation
of them.

I use the terms of consciousness and unconscious self,
for they are easy to understand, although the two terms
are not opposites.   It is difficult to express successfully
what one wants to express by means of words, and the
verbalism always falls short of what one would have it
express.   Consciousness can be expressed by social aspect
(of the psychic zone), a point on which Blondel (of Stras-
bourg) insisted, who, in his book on the *Morbid Conscience,*
has shown the importance of the social element in the
conscience of everyone.   One might almost say that our
consciousness results from our rubbing shoulders with our
social environment.   Montaigne in his day showed the
usefulness of rubbing one brain against another to produce
light.

On the other hand, the intimate aspect is that which is
turned towards the interior of the being, of which the
pathological form ends in the autism of the hebephrenic,
an autism expressible in spiral curves which tend to en-
croach on the centre.

This same distinction is found in Léon Daudet in his division of the " self " and the " me." The *self of Daudet*, which he exposes in his *Rêve éveillé* (Waking Dream), is consciousness ; the " me " of Daudet is the unconscious self. He showed that, in this unconscious self, it is easy enough to remove the last alluvial grains, to find all the engrams that result from hereditary qualities. It is incontestable that it is in the analysis of the unconscious self that one may find most easily the traces of ancestral heredity, which plays a rôle in the conduct of individuals and which has been marvellously exemplified in the *Ghosts* of Ibsen, an author who, with Shakespeare, has, possibly, best understood the importance of the unconscious self in human reactions.

But it was not necessary to wait for a Daudet or an Ibsen to express the qualities of these differences. Recently I have written a little work on the relationships existing between the *sympathetic* and the *tripartite soul*[1] according to the conceptions of Aristotle and Plato. It is certain that the consciousness corresponds to the Λόγος of the Νοῦς, Νοῦς corresponding to the intuitive intelligence, while the Θυμὸς corresponds to the affectivity, to the heart, and the 'Επιθυμία to the deep desires of the organism expressing themselves by the variations in the cenesthesia. The consciousness corresponds above all to the Λόγος, that is to say the expression by the spoken word, by language, of the discursive intelligence. It is interesting, in this connection, to find the same ideas in the beginning of the Gospel according to St. John, in which it says : " In the beginning was the Word, and the Word was God . . ." a phrase which has been distorted by Goethe in the second Faust, where he says to the contrary : " In the beginning was the action . . ."

From the point of view which interests us, the consciousness corresponds principally to the Λόγος, while the unconscious corresponds principally to the Θυμὸς.

[1] Laignel-Lavastine, " Le sympathique et l'âme végétative," Société française d'histoire de la médicine, Nov. 13th, 1926.

If we pass from Hellenic philosophy to the philosophy of the Middle Ages, we find the same distinction expressed as clearly by the German Mystic writers öf the fourteenth century : in Suso as in Tauler or Meister Eckart, who taught at Cologne, one finds the distinction of the *ratio* and the *mens*, the ratio corresponding to the discursive intelligence, the mens corresponding to the unconscious self.

Now, it is rather quaint to note that this distinction, which has become a classic in theological teaching, has been taken up again as something new by certain disciples of the super-realist school of André Breton. One of his emulators, to wit young Crevel, has recently given a lecture at Oxford on the mens and the ratio, in the course of which he smote the ratio, which has the great defect of being logical, hip and thigh, while he exalted the mens, showing the quantity of psychological dynamism it contains. You see, that our latest super-realists, who think themselves an advance guard, are only following the great German mystic writers of the fourteenth century.

Furthermore, this distinction between discursive intelligence and intellectual intuition is the basis of the Bergsonian philosophy, and it has been the merit of Bergson, who is, perhaps, one of the last descendants of the great prophets of Israel, to burst the low roof of Sorbonne philosophy, which has lasted some thirty years, and to have enabled us to see through the hole the blue of the sky and aeroplanes, that go very high up, and sometimes too high.

This term *intuition* has had a great success, all the greater the more difficult its meaning has been to grasp ; how many pretty ladies have we seen who had the impression that they were intuitive, considering men as incapable of having intuition and leaving them only intelligence. They are unaware, however, that a distinction must be made between the two varieties of intuition, and that the intuition of Plotinus must not be confused with the intuition of Descartes.

Descartes' conception of intuition is purely intellectual, while that of Plotinus is more than anything else affective. But it is not purely an affective intuition, and here we find the defect of discrimination, of specialization, because the further we go into the unconscious self the less specialization do we find.

The divisions, which we arbitrarily made between intelligence, affectivity and motivity, are didactic divisions. All the psychic currents in our psychology have affective, intellectual, and motive charges, and it was the merit of Paulhan, that distinguished mind, a little too subtle perhaps to have all the success he deserved—for when you are too sincere it is hard to be successful—that he showed that the various charges of the psychological manifestations are found distinctly in the instinct of the unconscious self in the Plotinus manner of thinking— a little perhaps, I ought to say, in the Bergsonian view.

It is much the same division, but taking its stance chiefly on the viewpoint of the emotive manifestations, that we find in the religious sphere. I shall not recall to you here the parable of Jesus of Martha and Mary, in which Martha expresses the activity of the conscious and Mary the meditation of the unconscious self. Claudel has come back to this division, in exposing, in detail, the somewhat noisy activity of the *Animus* that busies itself with all sorts of things, and the concentration of contemplative thought of the *Anima*.

One must of course admit that these synonyms that I have given you are by no means perfect.

In making use, thus, of these two orders of conceptions, we find on one side : consciousness, social aspect, logos of the nous, ratio of Daudet, Martha, Animus . . . and on the other side : unconscious self, intimate aspect, tumos, mens, intuition, Mary, Anima . . . and we confuse sometimes these two conceptions, the conception of dispersion with the conception of clarity. Now, precisely the value of the mystic meditation, which one also finds in the artistic meditation but less perfectly analysed, lies in showing that one must strive for unity by the light thrown on the unconscious self, and from the fact of the lack of differentiation of the unconscious, this intensity of concentration produces the appearance of an activity which the superficial self could not have produced.

This is a point of extreme importance for it allows the explanation of the purpose in the re-entry of God into the citadel, as contained in the last book of Izoulet. Indeed, it is thanks to the concentration of unknown forces in himself, that the individual is sometimes capable of heroic actions of which he would be utterly incapable were he to rely only on his consciousness. This was seen in the war, where under the influence of the enthusiasm bred in the defence of a menaced country, we saw dyed-in-the-wool internationalists fight like lions, thanks to their unconscious, dealing only in their abstractions at the conscious level ; and this shows the advantage of certain deep convictions, such as religious convictions, over philosophy, which resides on the surface of consciousness.

Methods of Examination.—I now come to the study of the methods of examination : *superficial methods* and *deep methods*.

The *superficial methods*—I shall review those very quickly. In the presence of psychological phenomena, one must always take into account the intellectual, affective, and emotive charges of each phenomenon under observation, for in each one there are these three modalities,

One must also take into account the *degree of synthesis* of the individual studied, this synthesis which is expressed by the personality produced by the activity of these two great functions, consisting of, first, the psychological tension, and second, the autoconduction.

Psychological tension is an extremely precise conception expressed by Pierre Janet and used by Bergson in his " *Elan vital* " ; it is a comparison with electrical tension. It varies according to the time and with the case and most psychasthenics express this variation of tension very well, when they say that they feel "as if they were in a dream " ;

" I see people as if I were not sure that they were real."
Indeed normal people may experience these phenomena,
when they are fatigued, for example. These variations in
psychological tension express what Janet has called the
" *function of the real.*" In all psychoneurotics this function
must be studied.

The method of estimating the strength of the psychological tension is to have them repeat some words several
times in succession, for example the word " manutention."
Generally at the end of fifteen or twenty times the subject
will in a way have exhausted his function of reality. He
has the impression that he no longer understands its
meaning and finds it strange and unknown.

Besides this psychological tension we have said that the
autoconduction has to be investigated. It is the function
which, one might say, is of the very greatest importance
to us in the psychoneurotic. It is the great synthetic
function of the being, of which the fragmentary expression
is *attention*.

Autoconduction has been described by Toulouse and
Mignard, my regretted colleague and friend. It consists
of applying the attention of consciousness to the different
sectors of the psychology. It is in a way the " telephone
exchange " of the psychological system. When one has
a good autoconduction one goes to sleep as soon as one
goes to bed ; as soon as one sets oneself to work, one is
" off," there is no " friction." But if one has a poor autoconduction there is difficulty in falling asleep, in thinking,
in changing the switch, there is a frictional difficulty in
getting under way, and when one has finished there is a
continuance of involuntary cerebration. This resultant
resonance is the condition of " *mentism.*" When the
phenomena of autoconduction become progressively
weaker, there occurs escape of automatisms. From the
fact that the ribbon, which binds up the psychic flowers
in the bouquet of the personality, tends to become loosed,
the flowers fall away from the centre, curving over more
and more, till they eventually fall. The individual is

then completely *scattered*. By such studies, then, one can estimate the variations in the personality.

But this is not all. One must study the most important psychological expressions in the primordial depth of the being, that is to say the *three instincts*.

I have already spoken to you of the *instinct of self-preservation*, which passes quite naturally into another instinct, for if in the amoeba reproduction is an excess of nutrition, this excess in more highly differentiated beings gives rise to the *sexual instinct*, which plays an enormously important rôle in the psychic life by its drive interfering with that of the instinct of self-preservation. Of this interference is born, indeed, many more or less complicated manifestations, more or less morbid. But this instinct, from the fact that it gives a greater scope to the instinct of self-preservation by, in a manner, its extension to other sympathetic beings, quite naturally gives birth to the *social instinct*, which is the third instinct.

All the disturbances of these three instincts must be observed in the psychoneurotic, and thus we finish with the superficial method to come to the *deep method*, which permits of the study of the most commonplace manifestation of the unconscious self. I refer to the *dream*.

But a distinction has to be drawn between the two great varieties of dreams : on the one hand there is what is the dream strictly speaking, the *hypnic dream*, the dream of sleep ; on the other hand, the *waking dream*, or reveries. One will then come to *onirocriticism*, which is the examination of dreams, which has at the present a second growth in favour, thanks to the works of Freud. I have recently published a critical and semeiological study of dreams which shows their incontestable value.[1]

It is also very important to analyse the reveries in their two main forms : on the one hand the *diffuse* and *spontaneous reveries*, and, on the other, the *systematized* and *orderly reveries*, focused on a point, such as Newton's reverie, the starting-point of great discoveries, for you

[1] *Journal médical français*, Nov., 1925.

know that without imagination and reverie discoveries are not made.

Parallel with the study of dreams, the study of *slips*—for instance slips of the tongue or of the pen, or slips in practical activities—is of considerable importance ; and in thus analysing individuals one often uncovers an unconscious that is endeavouring to conceal itself.

When one cannot have recourse to observation, one uses experiment and utlizes the *association-word test* of Freudian method. For this the subject to be examined is placed in a perfectly quiet room, and is allowed to develop as spontaneous a reverie state as possible. He is then given a certain number of words and is requested to express, as honestly as he can, the images that arise in his mind in response to these words. The reaction-time is noted as are vaso-motor or emotive reactions which may occur. I must say that it is chiefly when there is no reply that the best results are got. It is, indeed, when the association words find no echo in the conscious, that the *" water diviner "* of the *unconscious* becomes aware, if there are subterranean rivers, that the question is to make them come to the surface-level. It is a method of " flushing " or " putting up " the deep complexes, which play a considerable rôle in conduct and which often have an emotive origin dating back to infancy.

I am now going to apply these methods to the study of several patients :

First Patient.—Mlle. Violaine H——. This patient has a bad heredity ; a paternal aunt, melancholic, certified. Her personal history consists chiefly of a scoliosis ; and I want to draw attention to the frequency of scoliosis in the psychoneurotic. She became nervous in 1926. She was a school teacher and had to give up her work owing to the condition of her general health. At that time she had gastro-intestinal trouble. I want also to draw your attention to the frequency of digestive troubles in the psychoneurotic. Since then she had had alternating periods of calm, of fatigue, of depression, of aprosexia (wandering attention), obsession, mentism, and of auto-scopy.

From the somatic aspect, Violaine is a *longiform*. She is 175 cms. in height and weighs 58.6 kilos. She suffers from visceroptosis, of the stomach and bowel to a marked degree and in addition she has a dropped kidney on the right side. She also had a uterine retroversion that was operated on in 1921. She has attacks of muco-membranous entero-colitis, and you are aware of the frequency of these sympathetic reactions in connection with periods of depression in the psychoneurotic.

Actually her gastric troubles give rise to two kinds of pain : late pain with a feeling of slow digestion ; early pain sometimes taking on the character of cramp and which forces the patient to eat to ease herself. Towards half-past four in the morning she awakes with gastric pain and a sensation of hunger. At one time Violaine was under observation for pulmonary trouble, but she recovered. Her systolic and diastolic blood pressure is 13.5 and 8 respectively on the Pachon instrument.[1]

The tendon reflexes are present. The menstrual function has been diminished for the past eighteen months.

The sympathetic troubles are chiefly characterized by instability. The oculo-cardiac reflex is exaggerated ; on compressing the globe there is a slowing of the pulse from 19 to 12 beats per quarter minute, or 28 beats per minute. The solar reflex is positive. The urinary pH is materially raised. This is a very important point ; it has risen to 7.8—indicating an alkalinity related to a blood alkalosis, which corresponds very well with the definition which my friend Cornelius and I gave [2] of anxiety, when we called it an *alkaline neurosis*. The cenesthesia of Violaine is characterized by an exaggeration of internal sensations, which are disagreeable and difficult to define, in the region of the osseous system and its nerves,

[1] See footnote on p. 44.
[2] Laignel-Lavastine and Cornelius, " L'hypoacidite ionique et l'augmentation des acides organiques, syndrome urinaire de l'angoisse," *Presse Médical*, 18th Nov., 1925.

F

particularly the ribs : she feels " them twisting round her body like a snake." The sympathetic chain feels to her like a " turning mass," and she says that she always has the impression that " she is a small person in a large body ; worked by muscles of iron."

The analysis of her unconscious indicates an asthenia, aprosexia, a state of anxiety, or that obsessive fear of death, and other sad things. Violaine always sees in her mind's eye the people she saw in the train on her last railway journey, and for a whole year she has heard the rumble of the train. In fact she hears all day the sound of her bath, when she has had one in the morning : thus she has poor autoconduction. She shows " *mentism* " : when she has been writing letters she constantly is recalling words she used, she repeats several times, for example, the words : " this ought to be known and told, told and known. . . ." She has *premonitions*, a sort of intuition, which foretells what is going to happen, in quite a vague but still striking fashion. She predicted the departure of her brother for Syria. Now, at that time he was at Dunkerque, and surely enough he was later sent to Syria. When in the country she said : " there is iron in this ground," and indeed there were ore mines in the vicinity.

She shows the phenomenon of *resonance*, which belongs in the category of the manifestations of mentism. In her unconscious, one distinguishes three main complexes : mystic crises with a state of doubt ; a need to devote herself, to have some living being to cherish, which last led her to an episode that lasted some time and of which she still suffers the painful aftermath ; lastly she has a hate, and a very lively hate it is, for her mother-in-law.

The study of Violaine's dreams have a certain interest, for, being an educated woman, she has been able to furnish us with very explicit information. She dreams in spite of what she calls unbroken sleep. She has difficulty in falling asleep when she goes to bed. When she dreams, the dreams do not wake her, she is completely unconscious, and she adds that she feels soothed by her dreams.

In this we see the cathartic function of the dream. This feeling of being comforted derives from the fact that, in her dreams, she " fatigues herself physically," as she terms it ; and this is extremely important and I want to emphasize this comfort, which the patient experiences in her sympathetic field, by diverting the nervous influx into motor channels. This shows the unwisdom of the behaviour of M. Bergeret who, finding his wife in intimate conversation with M. Roux, merely picked up the *Revue des Deux-Mondes* instead of letting fly at the people in the stage box ! And I want to impress on your attention the *staircase-dreams*. The patient dreams of a staircase with enormous steps, of fantastic dimensions, like the stages of the Eiffel Tower. These steps show the void behind her, and she says that " she has to climb them and make other people climb them . . . and that she wakes up at the bottom of the staircase." She was given androstine for this, with much benefit. I shall develop more fully, elsewhere, the significance of this oniro-therapeutic fact.

The point of this observation, that I want you to remember, is that here is an extremely complex case, who responded perfectly to the concentric method, of which I have talked to you. In addition there is a very interesting episode in her history. She had an affective transference to a young man, whom she loved platonically, and there was a coincidental relationship between this and periods in which she showed manifestations of mystic emotions, a point which was delicate to study but which, beyond all doubt, was of the first importance. The best way of indicating how the analysis of these religious states should be handled is to describe in a few words the different degrees which one recognizes in the spiritual state.

An analysis of the unconscious, which has been marvellously carried out by the mystics, must be our guide in discriminating between many states : whether they be æsthetic states, or psychoneurotic states. But in order to be able to orientate oneself in the descriptions given by mystics, I must remind you that a distinction must be made between the three essential degrees : the *purgative path*, the *illuminative path*, and the *unitive path*.

The *purgative path* consists in the suppression of exterior states, purgation first of emotions and of current sentiments.

In the *illuminative path* the synthesis becomes more limited, one tends towards unity.

In the *unitive path* the mystic unites himself with God.

These three states are found in the great mystic-writers, and the one who has given the best written description of these states is St. Theresa in her "Autobiography " and " Castles of the Soul."

St. Theresa of Avila described the purgative path in the first two abodes, the illuminative path in the third. The fourth abode or prayer of quietude corresponds to the state of passive prayer, which is characterized essentially, as St. Theresa says, by sleep, then by disappearance of the discursive intelligence in order to leave the foreground to intuitive intelligence. The unitive path is characterized by the fifth abode, which is the union ; and lastly the sixth abode corresponds to the transforming union.

I have begun by quoting St. Theresa to you, although she is indeed the last of the great mystic writers, who has given a good description of these states, because she has given the most complete description. But it is necessary that I go back to the beginning and speak of the Augustinian inspiration.

St. Augustine went very deep into the mystic life, a fact which one would never suspect in reading the St. Augustin of Louis Bertrand, who is entirely aside the point in this as he is in his criticisms of the medical profession. St. Augustine expresses the purgative path by the *virtus*, the illuminative path by the *tranquillitas*, peace : " I give you my peace " ; the unitive path by two degrees : *ingressio in lucem* (the entry into the light) and the *mansio in luce*, the abode in the light.

We find almost the same division in *St. Thomas Aquinas*, but expressed by adjectives instead of nouns. He divides the mystics into : *incipientes* (beginners), *proficientes*, those who are already in the illuminative path, and the *perfecti*, or those who have achieved perfection.

A mystic who makes a great appeal to me, because he began by studying medicine in Spain, and utilized his former clinical habit in the experiment of introspection, is *St. John of the Cross*. He describes the illuminative path under the title of the " *night of the senses* " and the unitive path by the name " *the night of the spirit*," but as the night of the spirit is only the night from the point of view of the discursive intelligence, and is actually in full light, it is a night which has that subdued light which is shed by the stars and corresponds to the intuitive intelligence.

Now one can make a large number of concrete applications of all those states, and it is precisely what Pierre Janet has done in a book, published by Alcan, entitled : " *De l'angoisse à l'extase.*" But you have not finished with the mystic states if you content yourself with the analysis of the positive states only. There are also to be studied the *negative states*, which throw light on the depressive periods in the psychoneurotics.

These *negative mystic states* have been admirably described in religious manuals. There is first the *state of lukewarmness* which causes vomiting, then the *acedia*, which caused ravages in convents and whose most dangerous hour was the one which follows noon. It is the " Démon de midi " of which Paul Bourget wrote in his novel of that title.

Acedia is a variety of melancholy and languor, characterized by aridness and sadness of the spirit and of which the attenuated form is " drought." As one knows *drought* frequently occurs in mystic states, in fact there seems to be a sort of alternation between the states of drought and grace. There is no doubt that the variations of the state of grace deserve to be studied medically, for one can, in many cases, successfully establish a relationship between these variations and the variations in cenethesia. It is not my intention to discuss grace from the theological standpoint, but merely the psychic states, which very often would appear to accompany its effects.

I am not going to elaborate further a subject which merits, however, a large development. I only wanted to show that there are transitions between what we have been studying in the mystics, the patients in our wards, and what one sees in the artistic manifestations, especially poetry. L'abbé Brémond has shown that pure poetry is characterized by the trance. Whichever staircase one takes, whether poetry, literature, intellectual, æsthetic, or religious prayer, one always arrives at the same point, with the *trance*, a point which is the union between the divine and the human, passive contemplation, the fourth abode of St. Theresa.

Second patient.—Mme. Thomas is a case of doubt of the pure type. She has the great advantage of not dying of her literary efforts, as Seneca said. She is content to tell her story shortly and simply. She says : " I go and look out a pile of linen. I put it down, then I want to put it in my apron to take it to the wash, and I feel compelled to look around on the floor several times, to see if I haven't missed any. I know I haven't, but I feel forced, in spite of myself, to look around several times. . . ."

One could not express better, nor in a more striking way, obsessive doubt in all its purity, for the reason that this woman has no psychological cultivation. She does not interpret the facts. She gives them just as they are.

Third patient.—Mlle. Lab——. This patient has had nervous attacks. She says she has fallen down and struggled ; felt that something was choking her. The first time it happened she felt sad afterwards. This is relatively a common type of case ; a hysterical attack brought on by an attack of depression.

Fourth patient.—Mme. Tri——. She is obsessed. She states that when she was a child, one day, in the country, a serpent wound itself round her foot, and from that date on she has been nervous. An interesting point in this case is that she has manifestations of obsession by contrast ; she is a very worthy woman who is obsessed by a dog that once frightened her and of which she still has shameless and obscene visions, of which she refuses to give any details, and which appear to her especially when in church ; she is, I repeat, the type of contrast obsession.

Fifth patient.—Mlle. Bla——. She says she had been led to become a medium, but gave it up some time ago. She relates how, at one séance, she was deprived of her power of automatic writing, but that she has retained in herself the presence of a spirit that she hears ; and she complains of feeling electric shocks. She has been in this state since her menopause. From the fact that she was in a spiritualistic environment, she has symbolized her anxiety in the form of spiritualistic manifestations, and she has believed that she was possessed by a spirit. These are the symbolic manifestations that I wanted to show you.

Conclusions.—In the psychoneurotic there are psychophysical relations which show the necessity of my *concentric method*, that allows of placing the facts and arranging them in order.

In the second place, one appreciates the importance of the intermediate tendencies, the higher tendencies remaining intact and even serving for the symbolizing of the disturbances of the intermediate tendencies.

In the third place, one sees the value of the critical study of the different clinical complexes which one may uncover, because the manifestations, be they doubt, phobia, or ecstasy, do not always depend on the same mechanism. This is very important. I have shown you how obsessive doubt may terminate in very varied processes. And this again shows the usefulness of the concentric method in not attributing to the same pathogenic causes manifestations which may be similar in their expression, but not in their mechanism or in their pathogenic treatment.

In the last place, the necessity of establishing an *interzonal determinism* must be noted (that is to say between the different zones of the concentric method) and not a superficial determinism.

Indeed, the following is a frequent manifestation : certain individuals experience in fear, for example, a pleasure which may be accompanied by the loss of prostatic fluid. There is in this something that is surprising and which has been expressed in comedy. Molière makes Dorine say : "And if I enjoy being beaten ! " a thing which remains obscure in *plane psychology*, but which is well accounted for by the *diagnosis in depth*.[1]

Anxiety is a function of Vagus stimulation, and sex-pleasure is a function of stimulation of the pudic nerve. The pharmaco-dynamic reactions of the pudic and vagus are the same, the pudic nerve being a part of the vagal system.

One can thus understand that the intensity of the anxiety reactions should be related to the intensity of the excitation of the pudic nerve.

From this one can conclude the utility of always making a diagnosis in depth and not being satisfied with *plane psychology* ; and in fact one can say that to-day there are no psychiatrists, worthy of the name, who limit themselves to a single method of examination.

[1] Laignel-Lavastine, "Anxiété, volupté et pneumogastrique," *Paris Médical*, 18th Oct., 1924.

V

THE UNCONSCIOUS SELF OF PSYCHONEUROTICS, IN THE LIGHT OF ASCETIC AND MYSTIC EXPERIENCE

My dear President,

You have been too eulogistic of me and, I fear, after such an introduction, ladies and gentlemen, you will be disillusioned.[1]

Before commencing, I should like to thank Mlle. de Faissal, who is the moving spirit of this Maïeutique, the president of the society, and also Mme. Papillault, the vibrant poetess, whose words hold such charm.

Your high praise, my dear President, recalls to my mind that, if you have presented my *curriculum vitæ* in so sympathetic a fashion, it is because you are the colleague of two of my masters and friends, M. Pierre Janet and Dean Berthélemy. Your memorable work on Romanticism and its relations to Mysticism somewhat intimidates the physician that I am, especially in the rather delicate field that I am about to enter. But my hope is for your indulgence, because romanticism has accustomed you to the relativity of the contingencies of time and place. I also hope for your indulgence, ladies and gentlemen, in that you have come here this evening to hear me, for which I thank you warmly. And I count on that indulgence because I fear that I may disillusion you, for this reason. In coming to hear me deal with the subject of mysticism, as a medical man, you may have thought that it was my intention to treat of those theatrical

[1] Lecture delivered in debate, 7th April, 1927, to the Maïeutique, Baron Seillière presiding.

and somewhat dramatic manifestations that are of such popular interest. Such is not at all my intention.

On the other hand, you may have thought that I have been influenced in my choice of this subject by the well-merited stir caused by a book on St. Theresa recently published by one of our most brilliant Academicians. There is no connection. So, leaving for elsewhere my criticisms of this book, in which the author makes violent attacks on the medical profession, I shall begin my subject.

I exclude from the question the popular dramatic manifestations of certain mystics, the pathological troubles of certain others, and the study of the diseases of religious feeling, which were so excellently carried out formerly by the regretted Murisier.

I am going to talk to you on the unconscious self of psychoneurotics as illuminated by ascetic and mystic experience.

My first duty, then, is to define these terms before giving a schematic description of ascetic and mystic experience which will allow me to throw light on the unconscious of psychoneurotics. Thereafter, we shall draw some theoretical and practical deductions from this study.

I

DEFINITIONS

i.—*The Psychoneurotic.*

The psychoneurotics are difficult to define, because, in my opinion, the psychoneuroses are neither diseases, affections, nor syndromes. A disease is defined by its cause, an affection by the localization of the morbid process. and a syndrome by the appearance produced by the particular functional disturbance. The picture of the psychoneuroses is too complex and too changeable to be framed in one of these groups. In dealing with the psychoneuroses one must proceed by elimination as in the isolation of a salt chemically. These patients being practically intermediate between psychopaths and those suffering from organic affection of the nervous system, it is first necessary to establish limits both on the psychiatric and neurological sides. A psychopath, who is unaware of his morbid condition and out of touch with reality, is not a psychoneurotic. A neuropath who, according to the criterion of Babinski, shows physical signs of organic affection of the nervous system, is not a pyschoneurotic either. But there may occur in a psychoneurotic an associated organic nervous affection, and also many mental affections have a stage of psychoneurosis before their full development. The psychoneuroses, therefore, do not appear to me to be either diseases, or affections, or syndromes, but merely *evolutionary stages* of extremely varied affections.

The characteristic, then, of the psychoneurotic is that they do not show any physical signs of organic affection of the nervous system, are aware of their pathological state, and are not dislocated from their social environment. When one examines them carefully one finds absence of neurological signs in the sensory-motor system, but constantly finds signs of disturbance of the sympathetic nervous system ; and, furthermore, in these patients, there generally is found a lack of order between the various disturbances of psychic, nervous, endocrine, or visceral functions, which they present.

In my third lecture,[1] I showed that in order to diagnose psychopaths one had first to clarify the peripheral atmosphere of *psychic* and social reactions of the intimate life, to study the second nervous zone in its outer sensory-motor part and inner sympathetic part, then the *endocrine* zone, and lastly the *visceral* zone, to arrive at the centre or *morbific kernel*.

In the psychoneurotic, there is a mixture of sympathetic and sensory-motor nervous manifestations, and, in addition, the disturbance affects the *intermediate tendencies* of Pierre Janet ; the lower tendencies being often unaffected,

[1] See page 47.

as are also the higher and it is a characteristic of them that their point of origin is diffuse and that their end-point is in the ethic and æsthetic. It is the intermediate zone which is affected.

ii.—*The unconscious self.*

The unconscious self has long been known in religious literature, and it is curious to note that in classical literature it is a new thing of relative recency, Pierre Janet having first drawn attention to it in his thesis on *psychological automatism.* William James added much to our knowledge of the subconscious and Meyers, in his studies on the subliminal, has compared the human personality to an iceberg, of which the greater part is submerged in the sea of the subconscious, while the upper part, shimmering in the sun, corresponds to the consciousness.

This organic self Clemenceau[1] calls the " clair-obscur " of our ancestral emotivities.

iii.—*Ascetic and Mystic Experience.*

The ascetic and mystic experience is a fact ; those who practise it have the impression of experiencing God.

Before making a distinction between the ascetic and the mystic experience it is necessary to define those two terms.

The ascetic, ἀσκητὴς, the man who practises (ἀσκέω, to practise) is he who consecrates himself by piety to mortifications. The ascetic experience is that of the man who devotes his attention to the virtues and the means of acquiring them. The mystic, μυστίκος, μυστὴς, the initiate, is for Littré he who refines devotional and spiritual things. More properly (from μυέω, I initiate, I grasp, I form), the mystic is he who has a character of allegorical spirituality. (Littré.)

This term of mystic is very much used by doctors, writers, and other people in a variety of senses.

[1] Clemenceau, *Au soir de la pensée*, t. i, p. 24.

In medicine, *mystic delirium* is the same thing as religious mania, and when, clinically, one speaks of a mystic one means by that a patient whose trouble has a religious tint.

For writers, the mystic is most often a person who is very passionately attached to a divine or human ideal, *passionately idealistic*, who cannot explain clearly the high causes of his passion. If he is called mystic it is because of this mystery, this obscurity, and this intuitive and incommunicable knowledge.

Other people use the term mystic to describe anyone who is an enthusiast, hard to understand, living in a fashion unlike his fellows, and who prefers dreams to realities. Thus it may be used of an enigmatic writer or a utopist preaching a social or æsthetic system. The rationalist school of Cousin considered the Christians mystics because they admit of the supernatural. This change of denomination allowed him to attack Christianity without appearing to do so too obviously.

To-day, many philosophers class as mystics all Christian, Buddhist, or Moslem ascetics, when they manifest a strong religious feeling and the desire to find unity with God.

The mystic, in the wide sense, is, I should say, a *passionist of faith*.

But, in the narrow sense, the mystic is one who is shut in, secret. One must keep in mind the connection of the word with the *mysteries*, the secret cults of polytheism.

From the Catholic viewpoint : A. Poulain in his *The Graces of Prayer*, characterizes as mystic the *supernatural acts or states, which our continual striving or endeavour cannot successfully produce*, even in slight degree or for a momentary time. " Ordinary prayer," he writes, " may be compared to the atmosphere which encircles our earth. Birds fly through it at their will. But this atmosphere has its limits. Above these, the birds, do what they may, cannot penetrate, even though they double their efforts

God alone could carry them there. This upper region where the wing is of no avail, is like unto the mystic state."

Passive state is, then, synonymous with mystic. In illustration here is a confession of a spiritual soul : " I imagined that I had the supernatural at my command. Then, for quite some time, I gazed with fixity upon the Holy Sacrament during the Elevation, naively begging it to show to me the face of Jesus on the Host. I wished for that with such intensity, and, as at that time the Good God accorded me all things, I did not understand that he might withhold me that. By dint of staring, with the good eyes that I had then, I managed to make out the Cross of the Agnus Dei stamped upon the unleavened bread, but never the adored features that I hoped to see miraculously engrave themselves upon it. I came away disappointed and with eyes smarting from the flickering of the candles. Later on, I understood that my conduct had been reprehensible, and I asked the forgiveness of Our Lord. But if, by dint of auto-suggestion, I had succeeded in seeing what I desired (at that time I was nervous in no small degree) all my spiritual life would have been falsified, for I should have believed, as many naturalists do, that the supernatural inevitably flowers on a natural ground prepared and ripe for its reception, whereas there is none such. Daily I see that the divine is not at our disposition outside of grace, that it is supernatural, absolutely separate, objective, yet perfectly adaptable to all."

This definitely shows the mystic fact as passive, infused, free. It is, as Huysmans said, the irresistible entry of an outside will into one.

Its apparition, often fortuitous, unhoped for and startling to the recipient, characterizes the *passive prayer*.

Let me recall to you that *orison* (oratio, orare, to speak, from os, oris, the mouth) is the synonym of prayer. Prayer is vocal or mental. The *mental orison*, which is made without words, is a contradiction in terms from the etymological point of view ; but words are like coins, whose current usage is independent of the effigies struck on their face.

This passiveness in mental orison appears like a grace. Indeed *grace* (*gratia, gratus,* agreeable) is what is accorded to someone as being agreeable and useful to him, without, however, being strictly due to him.

Let us now take up our place as clinicians facing the theologians.

Garrigou-Lagrange, in his *Christian Perfection and Contemplation,* gives very clear definitions from the Catholic viewpoint.

Theology is the science of God. It is divided into natural and supernatural theology.

Natural theology is theodicy (attributes and justice of God).

Supernatural theology is revealed theology. It n turn is composed of two parts : *dogmatic theology,* which is the studies of the mysteries, and *moral theology,* which deals with human actions, precepts and revealed counsels, grace, Christian, theological, and moral virtues, and the gifts of the Holy Spirit.

Ascetic and Mystic theology is only one department of moral theology.

Ascetic and mystic theology is only an application of moral theology to the direction of souls towards a more and more intimate union with God. It studies the laws and the conditions of progress of souls towards perfection. In the *ascetic part,* it is concerned with the virtues, criticizes their nature, their varieties, the means of their acquisition, the obstacles, the exaggerations and imitations to which they are susceptible. In the *mystic part,* it is concerned with passive states and infused virtues. The point of contact between the ascetic and mystic theology is in orison (prayer) when the *passive* state appears. Ascetic theology deals with orison as does mystic theology, but by convention it restricts itself to *ordinary orison,* that is to say, that which, like the non-infused virtues, depends on man's work. Thus the *Imitatio Christi* is an ascetic work, while on the other hand the *Castles of the Soul* of St. Theresa, from the *fourth abode* onwards, is a mystic work.

The mystic theology thus delimited includes itself two modalities. *Doctrinal mysticism* describes the soul seeing and tasting the mysteries, living in the so-called continual union with God. *Experimental mysticism* describes, for its part, " the loving and pleasing, entirely supernatural, infused knowledge, which alone the Holy Spirit can give us, by its unction, and which is the prelude of the beatific vision." The study of experimental mysticism, therefore, comprises two methods : the *deductive method*, belonging to the theologians, and the *descriptive method*, the only one which the profane may use.

I shall leave to the theologians the deductive method and I shall confine myself exclusively to the *descriptive method of experimental ascetic and mystic theology.*

iv.—*Illuminated.*

I must now explain the term *illuminated*. I say that the mystic experience illuminates the unconscious self ; I do not say that it explains it. Indeed, I am not going to seek information on the mystic states from pathological experience. I am doing just the opposite and I have chosen the mystics rather than the literary writers or the poets, as M. l'Abbé Brémond did, because they pass their life in that search which is the *raison d'être* of their existence, because their chief effort is directed to succeed in apprehending the divine, and because it is in this that I have the best chance of reaching a sincere description of their state of soul.

But I insist on the importance of the conclusion of M. l'Abbé Brémond in his " Evolution of Religious Feeling in France." His study of the great mystics of the seventeenth and eighteenth centuries showed him the extremely close relationship that there is between poetry and prayer.

II

SCHEMATIC DESCRIPTION OF THE ASCETIC AND MYSTIC
EXPERIENCE

This will be a short schema, which will serve as a basis
on which to build.

i.—*The Ascetic Experience.*

The *ascetic experience*, that is to say, the experience of
the ascetics before passive orison, or fourth abode of
St. Theresa, is first of all the *prayer.* It is evident that
prayer already permits an ascetic experience, a fact that
more or less all the faithful know. One must pass above
vocal prayer, keeping in mind the usefulness of the advice
given by St. Ignatius Loyola, in his " Spiritual Exercises,"
in which he insists on the importance of variations of
respiratory rhythm in obtaining an affective state in
keeping with the words.

In addition I evoke a personal memory. Six weeks
ago I was at Manrese, in Catalonia, in the church built on
the grotto of St. Ignatius. There at sunset, in contemplation of the rays of the declining sun illuminating the
yellow river and the mountain of Monteserrata which
loomed violet against a green sky, I understood how
Loyola had been able, in such surroundings, to find
inspiration in nature and rise to the state of passive orison.

But, apart from mental prayer, there are a certain
number of procedures which facilitate contemplation,
amongst which I would emphasize the importance of the
chaplet, which I frequently call the staircase of prayer.
Indeed, St. Dominic, when he invented the Rosary,
must have felt the existence of the unconscious self,
which needs to be dissociated from reality by a rhythmic
activity to enable it to submerge itself more deeply in
contemplation.

In addition the liturgy, with its chants and postures,
has a very important function, as has also fasting. The
fast is found in all religions, and rightly so, for it is more

G

than a mere hygienic measure. If one studies the curve of vagus excitability in its relationship to that of the orthosympathetic during the twenty-four hours, towards the end of night, when dawn is at hand, there comes what the Book of Job calls " the hour when man dies." Why ? Because vagal excitability is then at its height. You are aware of the importance of this excitability in the determining of the sentiments. Fasting increases vagus excitability, while eating diminishes it. Clinically, one notices that the escape of the different parts of the psyche from consciousness occurs in an individual with greater ease the more marked his vagus excitability is.

The religious teachers had already appreciated the usefulness of the fast in the facilitation of prayer.

This brings me to *fervour*, the variations of which have a relationship to *grace*, grace which, from the symptomatic point of view, may be considered as the highest point in the affective order.

Thus prayer appears to me to be a surge of the instinct of self-preservation, of which the high-point merges in the social instinct sublimated in God. As a friend wrote me : " The further I advance in prayer, the more I find a lack of differentiation completely filling the affectivity from which proceeds a firmer will to conform to charity. I do not yet find there the Platonic Νοῦς." In this sublimation of merged instincts readily appears charity, this illuminating and unifying love, which can fall on society as a rain of altruistic activity, with an intensity of enthusiasm, of which deliberate reason is incapable. Thus there becomes evident the superiority in social action of religion over philosophy. According to this conception, religion would appear as the symbolization of the supraliminal eruption of the unconscious, rationalized and accepted by consciousness.

As L'Abbé Brémond has said, there is, in the consciousness of the passivity of the mystic state, something which is found, not only in the mystics, but also in the philosophers and poets. They all express themselves in the same way ; they have the impression of a force stronger than they. One can explain it, from the psychic point of view, by a comparison with the subterranean rivers studied by Martel. There is a moment when the subterranean currents can come to the surface of consciousness ; the individual has the impression that this comes to him from without, when actually it is an irruption of the unconscious into consciousness.

From the practical viewpoint, whether it is a question of mystics, savants, or poets, certain people, under the influence of the intensity of contemplation, are capable of rendering services, in social life, infinitely more useful than if they were only served by their consciousness and discursive intelligence.

This statement of fact cannot be denied. The social value of the mystic state is clearly evident in itself. It is not for me to discuss here the divergent interpretations which theologians and rationalists put on it. Furthermore, in certain states characterized by the belief of the subjects in their passivity, even to admit the existence of the supraliminal eruption of their unconscious producing charity, would not be, necessarily, contrary to the religious point of view, for God exists in every human soul. I therefore end this paragraph with this phrase of Segond, the excellent pupil of Ribot : " In the total subconsciousness of the life of prayer, the perfect communion of the mystic soul with the inexhaustible source of personal autonomy and universal charity, becomes a reality by the constant vigilance of attention."

ii.—*The Mystic Experience.*

The *mystic experience*, which I realize I have already mentioned in anticipation, does not only comprise *positive states*, or states of grace. It also consists of *negative states*, sadness and drought (which I find so often in the souls of those who consult me) and which may terminate in the *acedia* of the cloisters, in the *Dêmon de Midi* of Paul Bourget, and in a multiplicity of temptations.

The analysis of the negative states would lead me too far from my subject so to-day I leave them alone. However, I shall deal with the *positive states*, that is to say, the *graces of orison* (prayer). Schematically, *vocal* orison is followed by *mental* orison and *passive* orison. St. Angela of Foligno has given a remarkably clear description of this progress upwards : " The orison," she says,[1] " is where God is found." " And there are three schools, or three parts of orison outside of which God is not found."

Actually there is *corporal*, *mental*, and *supernatural* orison. " *Corporal orison* is that which is performed with the sound of words and corporal exercise, such as genuflexions. This form I never give up. For this reason, indeed, that sometimes I wished to practise the mental (orison), and several times I was undone by sloth and sleep and wasted my time. For which reason I practise the corporal (orison). And this corporal (orison) leads to the mental. It should, indeed, be performed with great care, and when thou sayest : Our Father, consider what thou sayest. Not in haste, compelling thyself to perform a certain number in the manner of women who work by the number of pieces they make.

" It is *mental* when the meditation on God so fills the soul that it thinks of no other thing but God. And if some other deep thought enters the spirit, I call that also mental. *And this orison silences the tongue*, for it cannot speak. The soul, in sooth, is so filled with God that it cannot be occupied by any other thing than by thoughts or words of God or in God. And by this mental (orison) one comes to the supernatural.

" I call *supernatural* that orison in which the soul is ravished by this *pity* of God and meditation, so that it is lifted up, as it were, beyond its own nature ; and it understands of God more than it sees or than can be understood

---

[1] Le livre de la bienheureuse sœur Angèle de Foligno du tiers ordre de Saint François, documents originaux édités et traduits par le P. Paul Doncœur, Art. cathol., 1926.

by its nature ; and it understands what cannot be understood by it ; for all that it sees and feels is above its own nature.

" Thus, in these three schools each knows himself and God. And that which he knows, he loves. And the more he loves, the more does he desire to have that which he loves. And it is the sign of the true love, that he who loveth transformeth, not a part, but all his self in the Beloved. But that this transformation be not continuous, and not endure, the desire takes the soul to search out all those ways by which it might be transformed in the will of the Beloved, in order to come anew into this vision. And it searches for that which He whom it loveth, loves. And God the Father makes for us a way by the Beloved, to know by his Son, who was the son of poverty, pain and scorn and true obedience. Now, as there be no greater poverty than not to know God (to wit, the pride by which fell the first man), he found another poverty which we must observe."

This ascent presents multiple degrees, from vocal prayer to mental orison, to active meditation, to the Augustinian contemplative meditation, to the active contemplation or third abode of St. Theresa, to passive contemplation or fourth abode of St. Theresa which is the beginning of the mystic life and to the last abode of the orison of union and the transforming union. At the threshold of the mystic life, to the orison of quietude by active and passive purifications succeeds passive orison in the illuminative path and unitive path. One must not think, however, that this schema is always followed. In the first place the three paths are not necessarily marked by the same orisons. Nevertheless, this general schema is useful in facilitating the understanding of the states of orison, according to the authors, and here is a reproduction of a *table of concordance of degrees of the spiritual life*, after Garrigou-Lagrange.

Souls are complex. One cannot limit them with catalogue labels. If we follow, step by step, the history of orison states, we see that St. Augustine had already described three types :

1. The *beginners* (*virtus*),
2. The *progressing* (*tranquillitas*),
3. The *perfect* (with the two degrees : *ingressio in lucem* and *mansio in luce*).

Denys describes successively the purgative, illuminative, and unitive paths, whereas in the German mystics of the fourteenth century, Meister Eckardt, Tauler, and Suso, the illuminative path precedes the purgative. Thus, they describe successively the illuminative, purgative and unitive paths.

The passive purifications of the senses and of the spirit are already indicated by Gregory the Great. They have been very well analysed by Tauler and especially by St. John of the Cross. Here is how, in " The Dark Night," St. John of the Cross, who was not only a great theologian, but also a very good clinician and a marvellous poet, sings of the passive purification of the senses.

SCHEMA
OF CONCORDANCE OF DEGREES OF THE SPIRITUAL LIFE AFTER
GARRIGOU-LAGRANGE

		St. Thomas Aquinas.	St. Theresa.	St. John of the Cross.	St. Augustine.
PATHS	PURGATIVE	Incipientes.	SECOND Abode.		Virtus.
	ILLUMINATIVE	Proficientes.	THIRD Abode. FOURTH Abode. Quietude, Sleep of the Powers.	Night of the Senses. Deep Caverns of the Senses.	Tranquillitas.

PATHS (cont.)	UNITIVE	Perfecti.	FIFTH Abode. Simple Union. SEVENTH Abode. Transforming Union.	Night of the Spirit.	Ingressio in Lucem. Mansio in luce.

I

During a dark night,
Burning with a love full of inquietude,
Oh ! happy fate !
I went out unseen,
When my house was still.

II

Full of assurance in the shadows,
I went out disguised, by a secret staircase.
Oh ! happy fate !
In the darkness and secretly,
When my house was still.

III

Favoured by this happy night,
None saw me,
And I had eyes for naught.
Neither guide had I, nor light
Save that which glowed in my heart.

IV

This light guided me,
More surely than that of noon
To where one waited me
Who knew me perfectly ;
No one in this spot appeared.

V

O night that guided me !
O night kinder than the dawn !
O night that joined so closely
The Beloved to his Well-Beloved,
That gave unto the lover the lover transformed in him.

VI

On my bosom flower-covered,
That none else may approach,
He remained in slumber ;
And I, I welcomed him with joy,
And refreshed him with a fan of cedar-wood.

VII

The breath of dawn
Stirred his locks ;
And of his soft hand placed upon my neck
I felt the wound,
And all my senses in suspension hung !

VIII

My face inclined upon the Well-Beloved,
I there remained and I myself forgot ;
All ceased to be for me, and I myself abandoned,
Leaving all my cares
Lost amongst the lilies.[1]

In this state God begins to communicate, no longer by the senses as formerly by means of reason, but in a purely spiritual way in an act of simple contemplation.

It is the threshold of the mystic life, which corresponds to the fourth abode of St. Theresa. This orison is further often preceded by isolated acts of infused contemplation in the course of *Acquired Orison of Reflection* described in the *Path of Perfection*.

Now, let us continue with the detail of the Dark Night ; this staircase, which we find in the Dark Night of St. John of the Cross, as in the St. Theresa, always leads to

---

[1] Vie et œuvres spirituelles de l'admirable docteur mystique le B.P. Saint Jean de la Croix. Traduit sur l'édition de Séville de 1702, Publiée par les Carmélites de Paris. 6e. edit. Mame, 1922, t. III, p. 236.

humility, whether it be the twelve degrees of humility of St. Benoit or the seventh degree of humility of St. Anselme, it is always for the unitive life the development of the words of St. Paul in the Epistle to the Colossians (iii. 2-3).

" Set your affection on things above, not on things on the earth. For ye are dead, and your life is hid with Christ in God." *Vita vestra est abscondita cum Christo in Deo.*

Now, schematically, let me bring back to your attention the table of concordance of spiritual states (on pp. 86-87), in which is given, according to the different mystic authors, the progress from the purgative to the illuminative and unitive paths.

According to St. Augustine, the first degree is *virtus* and the second is *ingressio in lucem* and *mansio in luce.*

St. Thomas Aquinas describes in the purgative path the *incipientes*, in the illuminative path the *proficientes*, and in the unitive path the *perfecti.*

What is more important is to see the concordance between St. Theresa and St. John of the Cross. The purgative path corresponds to the first two abodes, then by the third and fourth abodes one reaches the illuminative path ; the unitive path passes through the fifth abode. In the seventh abode there is the transforming union.

You will notice that between the fourth and fifth abodes of St. Theresa there is inserted the *Night of the Senses* of St. John of the Cross, and that between the fifth and seventh abodes is placed the *Night of the Spirit.*

You appreciate the general outline of the schema of concordance of the different writers ; but it would be wrong to think that passive orison is always a definite limit between the ascetic and mystic parts of orison and the *Ascension of Carmel* would be unintelligible if we did not represent it to ourselves as a double rhythm, that, in many respects,is simultaneous,on the one hand the rhythm of active disposition, which may go beyond the fourth abode, and, on the other, the rhythm of passive purification, which may appear at certain moments some time before the fourth abode.

As Jean Baruzi[1] says, in his Sorbonne doctorate thesis on St. John of the Cross, the *incipientes* of St. Thomas have not yet experienced the night of the imagination. They are still *in the sensible plane*. It is not surprising that some are still bound to sensible orison. Thus, the night which is approaching is the night of the senses, and the orison, which this night will regenerate, is the sensible orison. Furthermore, there is no constant relationship between the value of our thoughts and the perfection of our spiritual experience. The history of the mystics is evidence of this. Also, according to St. John of the Cross, the dark night is destined to assure a relationship, which will be established in the depth of the being, between a theoretical exactitude and a sublimity of the action.

These considerations of the contingence of the states of soul in orison are very important. They show the *ascetic* and *mystic oscillations* of these states and it is only in this spirit, free of all rigid schematism, that one could follow the progress of the spiritual soul from the *Ascension* of *Carmel* and the *Dark Night* up to the *Spiritual Canticle* and the *Living Flame* of *Love*.

In this progress I could not choose a better guide than St. John of the Cross, who shows in his writings that he is a very shrewd observer of the states of orison. I think it likely that his years of medical apprenticeship developed his powers of observation. *Jean de Yepès*, the future St. John of the Cross, was indeed a hospital attendant, for some thirteen to nineteen years (from 1556 to 1562) at Medina del Campo, in the same hospital as Gomez Pereira and probably in his wards. I remember that it was in 1554 that the great clinician Gomez Pereira published his *Antoniana Margarita, opus nemque Physicis medicis ac theologis non nimis utile quam necessarium*, per Gometium Pereiram, 1554, Medina del Campo, which was the product of his long medical researches.

---

[1] Jean Baruzi, *Saint Jean de la Croix*, 1924.

I shall give five examples to demonstrate what I put forward : *the differential diagnosis of the states of orison and visions, the clinical analysis of shameful movements in the course of spiritual exercises, and the positive diagnosis of the infused character and of the three paths, in the natural and supernatural order, purgative, illuminative, and unitive.*

i.—*Differential Diagnosis of the states of orison.*

St. John of the Cross distinguishes three great causes of error, the unwholesome manifestations, the manners of the enlightened of the world and the " diabolical deceits."

Since orison is prescribed, he analyses the defects of sensible orison before dealing with the passive.

Sensible orison is renewed by the night of the senses, such is the fundamental idea. " The spiritual man," says Baruzi, " not yet purified, finds a sensible joy in religious exercises ; these are the long hours passed in orison, sometimes whole nights, the satisfaction derived from penances, fasts or sacraments. All that which the soul savours for the sensible pleasure it derives therefrom." There is, exactly, the general weakness that St. John of the Cross discerns in the " principiantes " and which he has closely analysed in the various expressions he uses in describing spiritual *pride*, spiritual *avarice*, spiritual *anger*, spiritual *gluttony*, and spiritual *excess*, to which I shall return later.

ii.—*Diagnosis of Visions.*

This diagnosis is clear both in St. John of the Cross and in St. Theresa. He distinguishes *exterior* visions, which correspond to psycho-sensory hallucinations, *imaginary* visions which correspond to the physic hallucinations of Baillarger, and the *intellectual* visions, abstract intuitive cognitions of all sensible forms.

iii.—*Clinical analysis of " shameful movements and acts in spiritual exercises."*

Louis Bertrand, in his *Sainte Terese*, writes (page 221) : " Either these two words, sexuality and erotomania, have no longer any meaning, or one has to admit, with what is common experience, that the least sexual emotion is absolutely incompatible with religious emotion."

You appreciate the dilemma ; now, one can answer that the two propositions do not correspond to reality. In the first proposition, there is a very great difference between sexuality and erotomania, it being understood that erotomania is a delirium of passion that is essentially platonic with a basis of pride.

As for the second proposition, I believe it indicates that the author, although he is an author, has not had as wide an experience as the religious or lay confessors. Let us confine ourselves to-day to the experience of a religious confessor.

Referring exclusively to the orthodox St. John of the Cross, I find the following in his *Edicion critica*, Vol. II, pp. 13-14 : " Porque muchas veces acaece que en los mismos ejercicios espirituales, sin ser en mano de ellos, se levantan y acaecen en la sensualidad movimientos y actos torpes, y á veces aun cuando el spiritu está en mucha oracion, o ejercitando los sacramentos de la Penitencia y Eucaristia " ; that is to say : " It often happens that, in the course of the spiritual exercises themselves, there occur involuntarily in the sensuality ' shameful movements and acts,' and sometimes even when the spirit is in full orison or during the sacraments of the Penitence and the Eucharist."

How is it that this occurs ?

St. John finds four causes :

1. First of all, it very often occurs because our nature finds pleasure in spiritual things. " Porque entonces el espíritu se mueve á recreacion y gusto de Dios, que es la parte superior; y la sensualidad, que es la porción inferior, se mueve á gusto y deleite sensual, porque no sabe ella tener ni tomar otro ; y toma entonces el mas conjunto á si, que es el sensual torpe " (p. 14) ; that is to say : "While our spirit moves towards the discernment of God, our senses move towards the sensual pleasures, because they

do not know how to have or acquire another (pleasure) and they take that which is the nearest at hand to themselves, that is to say sensual turpitude."

2. The second cause of these carnal disorders is the demon, which thus produces a weakening of the orison, a firm resistance against these disorders and there result all the stronger from this very fact vivid impressions "which are very ugly and very shameful" and which intrude upon the thought and spiritual things and upon the image of those who aid us in our inner life. " Y no solo eso, sino que llega (demon) á representarles muy al vivo cosas muy feas y torpes, y á veces muy conjuntamente acerca de cualesquier cosas, espirituales y personas que aprovechan sus almas, para aterrarlas y acobardarlas." One could not give a better description of the *contrast obsessions*, and St. John has perfectly grasped the fact that it is " this resistance to the disorders themselves " which strengthens them. He adds as a very sound clinician : " If such torments attack us, if by chance they affect a *melancholy temperament*, the violence of the obsession is extreme and as a rule only the dark night will enable us to overcome them " (pp. 16-17). I have seen, at the Laennec hospital, an elderly spinster, with symptoms of menopausal melancholy, whose contrast obsessions corresponded to the above description.

3. The third cause of these sensual torments is the very fear they inspire in us. He was referring to the multitude of the *scrupulous*, of whom St. John, as a director of consciences, had a large clientèle. It is unnecessary to emphasize it, it is such a commonplace. As a practical point, I have found, in St. Thomas Aquinas, from his very clear distinctions between the spiritual states and the bodily reactions, a very effective means of calming many of these scrupulous cases.

4. Lastly, St. John, carrying his analysis further, makes out in people who are " tender and fragile " a sensuality which is, one might say, to use Baruzi's phrase, co-extensive to emotion. In such, there is the addition

to every orison of the "spirit of indulgence," which "intoxicates" them, in such a degree that they are as if "buried" in the enjoyment of "this vice" and sometimes one notices that "depravities and rebellious acts" occur. The page is so important that here is the exact text in the *Edicio critica*, Vol. II, p. 17.

"Hay también algunas almas, de naturales tiernos y deleznables, que en viniendoles cualquier gusto de espíritu de oracion luego es con ellos también el espíritu de lujuria, que de tal manera los embriaga y regala la sensualidad, que se hallan como engolfados en aquel jugo y gusto de este vicio, y duro el uno con el otro pasivamente y á veces se echa de ver haber sucedido algunas torpezas y rebeldes actos."

All this proceeds from the very frailty of these natures, since the same effect is produced in them by anger or some other trouble:

"La causa es que como estos naturales sean, como digo, deleznables y tiernos, con cualquier *alteracion se les revuelven los humores y la sangre;* y muden de aqui estos movimientos, porque á éstos lo mismo les acaece, cuando se encienden en ira ó tienen algun alboroto penas" (*Edicion critica*, Vol. II, p. 17).

You see that St. John of the Cross had certainly noted that different emotions, due to the small number of reflexes that our poor body has at its disposal, were capable of producing analogous reactions.

He could not know the similarity of reaction of the *Vagus* and the *Pudic nerve* nor the excitability of vagotonics. But his clinical observations have for that very reason all the greater value. They illustrate the physiological theory, that I gave[1] in explanation of the relationships between sensual enjoyment and anxiety and even any very strong emotion, which affects the vagal system.

One can further enlarge on this question, but instead of seeking in the diagnosis in depth of psychic manifest-

---

[1] Laignel-Lavastine, "Anxiété, volupté, et pneumogastric," *Paris médical*, Oct. 18th, 1924, p. 311-2.

ations the histo-physiological cause of subtle distinctions of affectivity, I shall end this short study with two sentences from Baruzi which will give you pleasure.

" Let us do more than concentrate our vision simultaneously on a sensation and the mental disorder that is mingled with it, and let us reflect on *sensuality captured in its living spontaneity*, so that no impure image may soil it : the analysis of St. John of the Cross would appear from this angle extremely penetrating and to touch the fine points, almost unstudied, of a problem that has scarcely been begun.

" Besides the sensuality, whose end is sexual, there is a *sensuality* that one might term *diffuse*. Autobiographical literature, were it completely outspoken and sincere, would throw much light for us on this. Such writers, who never speak to us fully of their distress, have they not above all experienced this torture, that is inflicted by a strong sensuality that ends in neither the discipline of the ascetic nor in the joyous impetuosity of desire ? " [1]

iv.—*Positive Diagnosis of the Infused Character.*

St. John of the Cross makes this diagnosis on three signs which Jean Baruzi analyses as follows.[2] The first is a special drought, in which the spiritual, while not feeling a desire for the " things of God," does not take pleasure in things deriving in any other fashion. He hastens to add, however, that such a sign is still a superficial one and that melancholy may cause a general distaste. A second sign is therefore necessary. Our thoughts must be in God with loving care " ordinarily." Lastly, a third sign is given by the uneasy feeling that all use of discursive thought gives us, by the drought that encompasses our senses and powers the while is formed a world of thought we do not understand.

This analysis, by which St. John of the Cross shows us the signs which we must show to be sure of our entry into the passive night, is very deep. To the two signs of

[1] J. Baruzi, p. 586.   [2] Jean Baruzi, p. 589.

general dislike and nostalgic love of God, he adds a functional criterion : that we can less and less avail ourselves of speech. This is what St. Angela of Foligno had already noted from the onset of the mental orison : mental orison stills the tongue. For St. John of the Cross this third sign does not appear suddenly. The ground is prepared for it by the aggravation of symptoms included in the second sign. The drought, that bears us down, already evidenced by the second sign, reaches the unconscious self, which the dark night will purify. But, in general, at the same time as a drought and emptiness overpower the senses, the soul experiences this desire of "being alone and in quietness," "without being able to think of any particular thing or having the desire of thought." If the soul went to the end of what it feels, if it knew " how to ease itself "—" neglecting all interior and exterior work, without care of accomplishing anything then "— it would immediately feel " delicately " (delicadamente) the internal renewal that is taking place. A reconstruction which is, indeed, so delicate that the soul ordinarily is unaware of it, even if it has the desire to feel it. It is a new world that is created in the greatest inactivity of the soul. . .   The soul is in this state regenerated above our consciousness.

v.—*Positive diagnosis of the three paths, purgative, illuminative, and unitive, in the natural and supernatural order.*

I have already allowed myself to be led far away from what is, strictly, my subject. Therefore I cannot follow St. John of the Cross in this positive diagnosis, which would demand long development. I only recall to you that in practice the three paths, in the natural order, may be confused. This fact explains the variance in the order of the paths according to the different authors. According to St. John, in the natural order of things the three paths, purgative, illuminative and unitive, follow each other but not always in the same order. In other words, one cannot give a single description of the abysmal experience.

The contemplation of the lesser mystics is not knowledge. It only appears, says Baruzi,[1] " as an affective wealth, psychologically of importance. It would be unwise to seek its possible origin in a metaphysical direction. But St. John of the Cross—and this would apply to the greatest speculative mystics of diverse faiths—is not content with a spineless mysticism. Contemplation, as he conceives it, is, essentially, a knowledge—a general and obscure knowledge. It is therefore quite allowable to compare it with æsthetic contemplation, which, if it cannot be called obscure in the mystic sense of the word, is certainly according to its rhythm, which is not entirely foreign to the mystic rhythm, a *general* knowledge. But, while æsthetic contemplation most often completes, and certainly never suppresses, the analytic effort of the artist, the mystic contemplation would definitely ruin the meditative thought. However, the discursive conclusions were not devoid of efficacy. But they disappeared after the flowering of mystic contemplation. And they shall never revive to their previous state. It is certain, as in one of the most profound phrases of St. John of the Cross—in the " abyss of joy "—" everything else is absorbed." And consequently, speech itself is absorbed by contemplation : *but it is absorbed without knowing it.* And such indeed is the essential difference between the analysis that leads to æsthetic contemplation and the meditation that leads to mystic contemplation."

You see the advantage of as perfect a knowledge as possible of the three paths : purgative, illuminative and unitive.

If we want to draw deductions from these rapid analyses, we might say that the ascetic and mystic sensibility is like the microscope of cenesthesia.

All psychologists already recognize that religious experience is above all others the richest source of affective

---

[1] Baruzi, *loc. cit.*, p. 589.

H

wealth. But in religious experience, it is essentially the ascetic and mystic experience that furnishes us, by its very sublimation, with the most precious documents on the infinite nuances of the affective life. Also I believe that I am entitled to speak of a *mystic æsthesiometry of cenesthesia and of the affective life.* I mean by that the confessions of the mystic writers would often appear to be like *magnified microscopic preparations of the affective fuses, that are lit by the cenesthesia.* I am well aware that my regretted friend Mignard, in his thesis on *passive joy*, showed that this mystic joy would not appear to be conditioned by marked cenesthetic sensations and that it was as if it were the function of an absence of all bodily perception, but this very absence, or the belief in this absence, is still something, without counting that St. John of the Cross had well noted *las tocas de Dios*, the divine touches, so often felt in passive orison.

To sum up, the mystic state, in my opinion, thus amounts to the *knowledge arising from the passivity of an undifferentiated psychology as the source of energy.*

Orison, thus, would appear as an orientated, polarized, passionate, unified, more or less mono-psychic reverie, with a feeling of passivity, presence, or union.

This relative psychic undifferentiation does not permit of the classical distinction between intellectual, affective, or motor elements. It is an undifferentiated, passionate, psychic flux approaching the primitive prelogical psychic states, and which would appear to be, in the light of criticism from the human point of view, a state of regression. It results all the more readily in action the more passionate and less differentiated it is. And so we get the explanation of the apparent paradox of the great contemplative thinkers who at the same time were great social reformers. And further, this return towards an infantile psychology can be related to the words of Jesus : " Unless ye become as little children ye cannot enter the kingdom of heaven."

Lastly, this state is accompanied by a feeling of power, beauty and ease of action, well known in reverie, and which would appear to characterize the twilight of consciousness like the iridization at the periphery of lenses showing spherical aberration.

III

LIGHTS THROWN ON THE UNCONSCIOUS SELF OF PSYCHONEUROTICS BY ASCETIC AND MYSTIC STATES

I must first give you a rapid history of the ideas on the unconscious self before analysing it in the psychoneurotics in the light of ascetic and mystic experience.

A.—*History and synonyms of the unconscious self.*

This history, which should be both philosophic and religious, would merit a long treatment. I shall, however, be content to-day to give a list of synonyms which is certainly not a complete one.

When one speaks to-day of the unconscious self one is immediately found to be in disagreement with all the anti-religious thinkers. This shows that for many authors the unconscious self serves to reintroduce the infinite into the human soul.

From the purely psychological point of view, the unconscious self in a first approximation would appear as being neither the discursive intelligence, reason, nor consciousness. In my definition I have brought it closer to the subconscious, to automatism, to the subliminal. To Gaston Rageot, as to Julian Benda, in Belphégor, it is the unintellectual self. As one cannot make precise psychological distinctions without going back to the Greeks, let us remind you that Plato distinguished in the soul, Ψυχή, the Νοῦς, the Λόγος, the Θυμός, and the Ἐπιθυμία.

The Νοῦς characterizes man " who alone is able to raise himself to the contemplation of the intelligible." " Purely intellectual contemplation is always in the eyes of Plato," as the late Victor Brochard wrote quite some time ago,[1] " the most perfect form of life. Sentiment is only a means by which to mount to thought : it neither takes its place nor is its equal. . . . It is thought only that attains the absolute." Plato is a pure intellectualist. His Νοῦς, which is the intuitive soul, has become the Cartesian intuition. The Λόγος the rational soul, is derived from the Νοῦς, and is an instrument of intellect. The Θυμός, the irascible appetite, the humour, characterizes the animal. The 'Επιθυμία, the concupiscible appetite, the desire, is the whole soul of plants. This is the reason why it is still called the vegetative soul.

I have shown, elsewhere, that according to Galen,[2] the humour (Θυμὸς) occupies an intermediate position between the intelligence (Νοῦς) and the general sensibility (Επιθυμία).

On the other hand, my conception of the sympathetic[3] is easily reconciled with the Platonic idea of the vegetative soul.

The whole contemporary physio-psychological movement tends, on the one hand, to correlate the variations of affectivity or psychic humour with humoral changes in the endocrine and sympathetic fields, and, on the other hand, to recognize an affective basis in the majority of mental troubles that are characterized by intellectual symptoms. This is, only with greater precision, as I said, the idea of Galen, who considered that the Θυμὸς was intermediate between the Νοῦς and the Επιθυμία.

This light, drawn from Timée,[4] will illuminate our path to the unconscious self.

In the first place, the unconscious varies with the *author* and the *time*. Therefore, I shall first enumerate its equivalents according to the authors dealing with it.

[1] Victor Brochard, *Et. de philosophie ancienne et moderne*, Introduct. de V. Delbos, nouv. edit., 1926.
[2] Galien, *De l'utilité des parties du corps*, Trad. Daremberg.
[3] Laignel-Lavastine, *Pathologie du sympathique*, 1924.
[4] Laignel-Lavastine, " Le sympathique et l'âme végétative, *Bull de la soc. française d'hist. de la méd.*, 1926, p. 381.

According to Plato, it is in the first place the Θυμὸς, the humour, in distinction to the Νοῦς, which is the intelligence of man that has scarcely emerged from the Ἐπιθυμία; thereafter it becomes in cultured man the Νοῦς, or intuitive soul in distinction to the Λόγος or *discursive reason*. It is in this sense that the divine contemplation is summarized in the classical Νοῦς Νοήσεως Νόησις.

According to Descartes, who in this inclines to the Platonic view, the unconscious self corresponds to the intuition.

This intuition, which is purely intellectual, differs from the Bergsonian intuition.

The intuition of Plotinus and Bergson, which is mixed with Θυμός, is the opposite of the discursive intelligence.

The Latins, keeping the Greek division of Νοῦς, and Λόγος, which became the Word of Christian tradition, made a clear distinction between the *mens*, which was the spirit, and the *ratio* which was the reason.

This distinction was kept by the German mystic writers of the fourth century. Johann Tauler, in his *Imitation of the Unhappy Life of Our Saviour Jesus Christ* (Noel translation, 1914, p. 400), says distinctly : " The intimate union with God in faith and love is only possible in the depth of the soul, *in mente*." And Father Pierre Noel follows this chapter with the following remark : " Faith, which is its soul, life, and form, cannot be received, in principle, except in the depths of the soul, in the spirit (*in mente*) as an immediate and truly vital subject. The thinking reason drawing its knowledge from the senses and the sensible perceptions and being unable to acquire it elsewhere since it is bound to the organs (nihil est in intellectu quod prius non fuerit in sensu), reason cannot be the immediate subject of divine faith which must be produced without images. *A fortiori*, the senses show themselves to be completely lacking in power. . . . This immediate subject is, if I may say so, the angel which is in man and which has perceptions that man knows not. Faith, which makes him know God as He is, by the word of God, is one of these perceptions, of which reason is incapable."

While the Neo-Platonic mystics, Tauler, Eckardt, Denys, St. Bernard, distinguish thus between the *mens* or depths of the soul and discursive reason, St. Thomas with Aristotle only sees variations of intellect. The former conceive them to be two distinct levels, while the latter only see them as variations of lighting of a single light-source. The reason for this is that the Rhenish mystics have taken the aspects of their spiritual experience to be philosophical entities. St. Theresa, who remained in the descriptive plane, speaks of the sleep of the powers during the intense moments of divine union. This formula makes the mystic experience and the conceptions of St. Thomas Aquinas agree : this thing of infinite peace and radiance, which one finds in complete refreshment, is not a new soul nor depth of soul, but as one author wrote me, the supreme well-being of this soul, God its hidden but real guest. Instead of saying always : turn to the depths of your soul, Tauler could simply have said : Shut doors and windows and put out the lights that blind those who shine with the ineffable presence.

In the Latin course of mystic tradition, the *mens* certainly corresponds to the unconscious self. Thus St. François of Sales understands it when he speaks of the ecstasy at the far point of the spirit.

On the other hand, the *ratio* corresponds to the discursive intelligence.

It is remarkable to note that it is the *super-realists* who, with young Crevel, in a lecture that he gave in 1926 at Oxford, have come back to this distinction of the *mens* and the *ratio*. It is indeed interesting to see that these super-realists who, before the war, thought themselves at the head of a literary movement are merely following the movement of the religious mystics of the fourteenth century.

However, one must admit that, amongst recent French authors, there is one man who has marvellously penetrated the shadows of the conscience and therefrom drawn elements of the first order. I refer to Marcel Proust. And this brings me to the likening of the *unconscious self* to the *prelogical stage* of the spirit.

This *prelogical stage* persists in each one of us underneath the alluvial sand of our *social experiences* and our *rational activity.*

Blondel has very well contrasted this intimate aspect with the social aspect. Léon Daudet, in his *Hérédo* as in his *Rêve éveillé*, has similarly contrasted the " me," which is an organic hereditary synthesis, with the actual personal " self," that is woven day by day.

This is, with a religious nuance added to it, Claudel's distinction between *Anima*, the contemplative soul and *Animus*, the discursive spirit, a distinction which, in a poet, would seem to derive from the gospel account of Martha and Mary, contrasting the active life with the contemplative.

In the *Nouvelle Revue Française* of the 1st October, 1923, Claudel published his parable " to explain certain poems of Arthur Rimbaud." Brémond thus quotes it in his preface to the *Entretiens avec Paul Valéry*, by Frédéric Lefèvre, p. xlvi :

" Things are not going well in the Animus and Anima household, the spirit and the soul. The time has passed, the honeymoon soon over, when Anima had the right to talk freely as she wished and Animus listened to her enchanted. After all, is it not Anima that brought the dowry and kept the household going ? But not for long has Animus let himself be reduced to this subordinate position, and he soon showed his true nature, vain, pedantic, and tyrannical. Anima is ignorant and foolish, she has never been to school, while Animus knows a whole lot of things. He has read a great deal in books. . . . All his friends say that one could not be a better talker than he. . . . Anima has no longer any right to say a word . . . he knows better than she what she wants to say. Animus is unfaithful to her, but that does not prevent him from being jealous ; for, at heart he knows, very well (no, he has managed to forget it), that it is Anima who has the money, and that he is a waster and lives on only what she gives him. Also he is always taking advantage of her and tormenting her to get money out of her. . . . She stays silently at home cooking and cleaning. . . .

"At heart, Animus is middle-class, he has regular habits and likes to have always the same things to eat. But recently something very curious has happened. . . . One day Animus came home unexpected . . . and heard Anima singing all alone behind a closed door a curious song, one he did not know, of which he could not make out the notes, words or key, a strange and marvellous song. Since then he has tried to get her to sing it again, but Anima pretends she does not understand. She becomes silent when he looks at her. *The soul becomes silent when the spirit looks at it.* Then Animus resorts to a trick, he acts in such a way that she believes he is not there . . . little by little Anima is reassured, she looks, she listens, she thinks she is alone, and noiselessly she goes and opens the door to her divine lover."

This is passive orison, inspiration, the trance.

This distinction of Claudel's which the Abbé Henri Brémond utilized in his *Poésie pure* and in *Prière et Poésie*, is already in St. Theresa.

Indeed, in her *Autobiography* she says : " I know someone who, although no poet, improvised couplets full of sentiment . . . her spirit had no part in this." There, exactly, is Anima who sings her song behind the closed door, as Claudel has it, without the help of Animus. But prior to St. Theresa, who indeed turns round again a little further on, I have never seen anyone who considered the spirit as the bourgeois of the soul and the soul as the poet.

This interpretation, which has become one for *Animus*

and *Anima*, is contrary to the tradition followed by the German mystics. In all the mystics, as Father Noel very justly remarks,[1] " The spirit (*mens*) is the angel that is in man and which has perceptions unknown to man. The soul keeps its etymological sense and is as a consequence the animator of the organs." It is certainly in the same sense that St. Francis of Sales, in his *Traité de l'amour de Dieu*, speaks constantly of the extreme point of the spirit.

But let us return to the poem of St. Theresa. She sings :

> But that causes in me such a pain
> To see God my prisoner,
> That I die of not dying.

In this song improvised by her *Anima*, St. Theresa sees her God within her a prisoner. This does not contradict the St. Thomas theory of the simplicity of the soul, since the divine inhabitation would be sufficient explanation that, once the powers asleep, the senses stilled, it is the guest who takes up the bow to play, he whom Sully-Prudhomme calls the Stranger.

> I list to a sublime Stranger weep within me
> One who has always hidden his land and name from me.

Thus the poetic trance touches the mystic trance.

It is the theory of pure poetry of Abbé Brémond.

One must not confuse the dispersion of conscience with its radiance. This is a point on which St. Thomas insisted in showing very clearly that the unity of the conscience obtained by the concentrated enlightenment of the deep Self augments the original tendencies. The light that is concentrated on the very centre of the soul by that very fact renders the peripheral parts less clear ; there results from it a sleep of the powers, a closing up of the senses on the exterior world, a dislocation of reality. This distraction recalls the schizoid state, but the resemblance of aspects does not imply identity of cause. The distraction of an Archimedes is not identical with that of a schizo-

---

[1] P. Noel, *loc. cit.*

phrenic. " One can feel by this example of the unconscious self how closely the ideas of theology, that our
worldly century disdains with all the lightness of ignorance,
touch close to life itself."
That phrase is not mine, it is from M. Gonzague Truc,[1]
a pupil of Ribot, in a book on Grace, published by Alcan.

B.—*Analysis of psychoneurotic states allied to the ascetic
and mystic experience.*

It is in scrutinizing the auto-observations of psychoneurotics and the diaries of mystics that one would find,
a priori, the necessary documents of this analysis.

I can only indicate the chapter-headings of this here
and dwell a moment on certain feelings, to which one can
easily find corresponding feelings in the works of *religious
intimate writers*.

Take first *Depression* with its many shades of degree, and
of which one meets marvellous descriptions in the *luke-
warmnesses* and *droughts* of the pious souls.

Then take the *Obsessions*, whose importance is so great
in the religious life that many of the *scrupulous* require
for their recovery the collaboration of a priest and a
doctor. Without emphasizing the interest of the *Acedia*
of the cloisters, the inspiration of Bourget's *Démon de
Midi*, I shall content myself with quoting this classical
description of temptation from the 13th chapter of the
1st Book of the *Imitation de Jesus-Christ* : " First a
simple thought is offered to the spirit, then a vivid
imagining, then a delectation and consent. So the enemy
invades the soul little by little when one has not resisted
from the start." One could not give a more perfect
description of obsession.

The *feeling of strangeness*, in relation either to one's
self or others, such a frequent symptom in fatigued people,
is often noted by mystics. The feeling of strangeness of
body may go as far as to create an impression of *lightness*,
of immaterialness, which would appear to be due to

[1] Gonzague Truc, *La Grace*, 1918.

modifications of cenesthesia.   In the case of *levitation*, the mystics lay stress also on these sensations of lightness, immaterialness, and absence of all contact with the ground.

The description of the mystics of imaginary *visions* and intellectual visions is precisely the distinction between psycho-sensory hallucinations and the psychic hallucinations of Baillarger.   The mystic is constantly insisting that the divinity has spoken to him in spirit, without words, soul to soul.   It is only in exceptional cases that he has heard with his ears and seen with his eyes.   In this latter case one has to be sure as St. Theresa remarks, that one is not dealing with disease, and in the former one must think of the possibility of the phenomena of resonance, as in the *mentism* of fatigued individuals.

The Illusion of already having seen, already heard, or of having already lived, so common in psychasthenics, had in the past impressed Pythagoras and it appears to me to have been the origin of his conception of the immortality of the soul and of metempsychosis.   Since I am so definitely conscious of having lived this present moment and that it is not in this life, it must be because it was in another, and my soul which thus remembers it, then inhabited another being.

The belief in *psychic passivity*, which comes into the immense problem of *psychological automatism*, is the characteristic of the *threshold of the mystic life*.   All the descriptions of passive orison from the fourth abode of St. Theresa onwards abound in information of the highest interest on the *evasion of automatisms*.   Before or with the feeling of passivity there may appear the feeling of a foreign presence.   This *feeling of presence*, of such frequent occurrence in the illuminative path, may appear as an episode in the purgative path.   According to whether this feeling is accompanied by confidence or fear, there is the tendency to make one think that the presence is either holy or diabolic ; and, also, according to whether there is association of the feeling with sensory or cenæsthetic impressions, it tends to cause the realization of an exterior influence or an interior *possession*. On amplification, in the unitive path this may go as far as the *mystic marriage* and the *transforming union*.

These terms, which at first shock because our habits of mind make us take them in the too material sense, express the current ideas of the Pauline theology. Indeed does not one read in St. Paul: " It is no longer me, but God that liveth in me " ?

But according to my definition of the psychoneurotics, in these patients, matters do not go so far. More than feelings of presence or possession, they have the *feeling of influence*. This impression which is often very fleeting, is a secondary interpretation of the consciousness of evasion of automatisms.

One same characteristic is found in all these psychoneurotic states that I have just reviewed : they are all *depressive states*.

In contrast, if I remove, from these ascetic and mystic states that have just been dealt with, the very rare cases that are complicated by diabolic interpretations, they all account for themselves by an *increase in psychological tension* and a rise in psychic value of the individual.

C.—*Synthesis.*

Now I come to the synthesis by comparison of the resemblances and differences. The former are those of which I have just been speaking ; one may consider the mystic description as a microscopic preparation that enables us to see in the magnified state the affective modifications. But the differences have the advantage over the resemblances.

Here, then, is the difference. In the mystic, the depression of the ascetic exercise always terminates in a growth of the psyche by faith, in contrast to the psychoneurotics in whom there is a predisposition to doubt and anxiety disturbance.

D.—Theoretical and practical deductions.

Let us now see the theoretical and practical deductions that one may draw from this study.

First deduction : the neurosis is often a ransom of holiness, but it is not the whole thing.

Second deduction : there is a very marked distinction between the psychoneurotic phenomena and the mystic manifestations.

Third deduction : the unconscious self of the mystics is a normal unconscious self, even although the mystics may have abnormal manifestations in their consciousness. On the contrary, the unconscious self of psychoneurotics is a sick unconscious self. There results from this main difference that the hypervitality which the mystic receives in the passive orison, must be distinguished from what happens in the psychoneurotics and shows the necessity of psychotherapy by faith in the psychoneurotics.

The treatment of psychoneurotics must therefore, at least in part, be inspired by asceticism and mysticism.

I come now to the *theoretical deductions.* You see that, if we now take a very distant bird's eye view of these states from passive orison onwards, they appear to us as essentially as a lack of psychic differentiation, as a real spiritual bath, out of which the soul comes with increased energy, as the phrase of Aristotle, one of the most beautiful of antiquity, goes :

'Ευδαιμόνια ἐνέργεια ἔστιν.

Happiness is energy. Later St. Thomas Aquinas was to say " God is love, and love is joy " ; and Thomas à Kempis, " O Charity, who art God, make me one with thee in love eternal ! " This truth exists for all time everywhere. " Who knows his soul knows God," the great Arab mystic Yahya ibn Moadh al Razi[1] has for his part expressed it.

I end with a word on the practical deductions : to treat

[1] Louis Masignon, *La passion de Al Hosayn ibn Mansour al Hallaj, martyr mystique de l'Islam.*

psychoneurotics well it is necessary to have a single spiritual management (psychoneurotics must not pass through the hands of several doctors, they should have one only) ; regular habits, a rhythm of life in which the too great fluidity of soul of the psychoneurotic can mould itself, maintain itself and not constantly spill over ; a state of joy, calm, and tranquillity canalizing the diffuse affective flux into definite liturgic habits. And this shows the importance of the therapy on which Pierre Janet insisted : the *psychological medications* ; wiping out of the past, analogous to general confession ; that simplification of life recommended by Epicurus and Tolstoi ; lastly elimination of dispersion of the spirit. How I should take that advice !

I come to a conclusion which considerably overflows the premises : to rationalize in the light of consciousness the affective irruption of the unconscious self, it is in this, one might say, that there lies the synthesis of the two great human tendencies : the Dionysian and Apollonian, as Nietzsche said : the Pythian cult of Delphi and the Reason of Athens, the mystic flame of Asia diverted into the Roman furnace.

CONCLUSIONS

In *conclusion* I shall say :

1. The description of the unconscious self given by the mystic Christians has a great documentary value.

2. It throws more light on the unconscious self of the psychoneurotics than do the musicians, writers, classical poets and philosophers.

3. But the psyche of the mystics differs from that of the psychoneurotics in that it shows an increase and not a diminution in psychic energy. It is by this criterion that one may recognize it, a point on which St. Theresa insisted at length and it is useful in enabling one to eliminate the false mystics, who have been very numerous in all times.

4. This increase depending on faith, at least in part, there is reason to *place faith in the foreground of the treatment of the psychoneurotic.*

5. This faith, at the minimum, will be threefold : naturally *confidence* of the patient in his *recovery*, confidence in the *treatment* that is given him and above all confidence in his *physician.*

This last word is the spiritual essence that I offer you in thanking you for the pleasure I have had in laying before you at too great length—I blame myself for it— several too short ideas.

THE DEVIL AND THE PSYCHONEUROTICS

A LECTURE DELIVERED BY M. JEAN VINCHON, ASSISTANT
IN THE NEUROLOGICAL SERVICE

BEFORE starting on the medical study of the demoniacal psychoneurotics, we must summarize the conceptions of the theologians.

According to their ideas, the demoniac are divisible into two categories :

1. First the *obsessed*. They are those who suffer the persecutions of the Devil, either externally, or internally.

External persecutions are represented as blows,burns, and contacts ; the internal as troubles in various parts of the organism.

2. Besides the obsessed, whose personality suffers but remains intact, the Church recognizes the *possessed*, who, on the other hand, lose their own personality to a foreign personality which instals itself in them. Such persons are liable to strange actions.

To give you an idea of them, I shall read a few lines from the *Théologie morale* of Debreyne,[1] a theologian who lived at the time of Charcot. He was a physician as well as a Trappist monk and he made his observations from those two particular points of view :

" The characteristics that theology recognizes in this state (possession) are as marvellous —the speaking and understanding of languages that one has never learned, the discovering of things that are distant and hidden, the making use of a strength beyond his age and

---

[1] Debreyne, *La Théologie morale*, Paris, 1884, p. 277.

condition, as in the accomplishment of physical acts, or in supporting suffering, in a manner which physiology cannot explain. To this can be added the pride, which dominates the character of the possessed, and also the horror he feels for sacred things in general, and particularly the horror he experiences on contact with blessed objects, even though he may be unaware what these objects are. This may be a permanent state, but as a rule it occurs as crises or exacerbations of his symptoms.

" It is of importance then to be certain that these marvels, when one comes across them, are definitely real, and not the product of illusion or deception. . . ."

I ask you to keep well in mind the second part of the enumeration of the states of possession, for we shall meet it again in the description of certain pathological states.

These distinctions of the obsessed and the possessed are very different from those of psychiatry ; the patients with whom we shall be dealing are possessed, but of a particular variety of possession.

They manifest secondarily the nervous troubles, from which they suffer, by means of a collective belief in the devil, and not by a delirium ; they are therefore very different from the insane in whom delirium is an essential feature, this delirium remaining always personal, and modifying, according to the tendencies of the individual, the facts of the general belief.

The relationships between demoniacal states and nervous diseases have been known from antiquity. They were first studied by a physician at the time of the Antonins, Cœlius Aurelianus.[1] These studies were continued by the physicians of the Renaissance and especially Johann Wier, who seems to have been inspired by the writings of the Byzantine demonologist Psellos. The view of these latter was that the devil took possession of the imagination of individuals and gave them the illusion that terrifying things that happened about them were

---

[1] Laignel-Lavastine et Jean Vinchon, " Sémeiologie des démono-pathies en 1580," in *Archivio di Storia della Scienza*, March 1, 1924.

reality ; he also gave them diseases such as melancholy, which is different from the psychosis that we call to-day " melancholia." The old melancholy was an organic and psychic disease, characterized from the organic point of view by hepatic troubles, hence the name of melancholy (black bile). From the psychic point of view it was not really depressing as is the melancholia of to-day ; the subject of it had a lively sensibility. He was capable of remarkable intellectual qualities ; the old authors thought that many men of genius were melancholics.

The doctrine, which teaches that the devil takes possession of the imagination of people and gives them diseases, is still supported by a certain number of theologians ; but it is not for us to enter the discussion of that here ; we shall confine ourselves to the exposition of the different clinical pictures that we meet in our patients.

In them, we have to deal sometimes with symptoms of the *emotive series,* sometimes with symptoms of the *imaginative series.* These symptoms are more or less mixed in the various clinical pictures ; but, nevertheless, one may make use of them in the description of the three great psychoneuroses: emotive psychoneurosis, hysterical psychoneurosis, and neurasthenic psychoneurosis.

The first to which we shall give our attention is a particular form of emotive psychoneurosis. It is characterized by contrast obsessions, which recall the horror of sacred things described by Debreyne in his *Théologie morale.*

The contrast obsessions have been studied in the most complete fashion by M. Seglas in his clinical lectures, in certain pages which I shall summarize for you.[1]

M. Seglas' view is that, in these obsessions, the psychic dissociation is particularly manifest. The obsessing ideas contradict the individual tendencies of the patient. For example an impulsive homicide often comes to strike

----

[1] J. Seglas, *Leçons cliniques sur les maladies mentales et nerveuses,* Paris, 1895, p. 127.

people for whom he has the greatest affection. The
example, which he gives, is that of a young girl of neuropathic inheritance who, about the age of puberty, begins
by having religious scruples, then goes through a stage of
neurotic doubt and finally, obsessed by her unhealthy
ruminations, vows to become a nun. She improves for
two years, but her vow is not taken. At a certain time
her sister falls sick ; the patient suddenly gets the idea
that her sister has been stricken because she herself has
not accomplished her vow. She goes through a second
depressive period of scruples, doubt and uneasiness. To
try to remedy this condition she renews her vow and again
she improves. But she does not want to make her mind
up to enter the convent ; each time that she is about to
join the Carmelites, she is seized, in spite of herself, by
absolutely contradictory ideas, characteristic of obsessions
by contrast. She can only think of romantic adventures,
ideas of marriage, and she suffers at such times terrible
anguish.

The contrast obsessions become more marked when
she is in church, she feels herself forced to blaspheme,
to make irreverent gestures, to pull faces before the altar.
At confession, instead of humiliating herself, she has the
desire to tell all sorts of things to make herself interesting.

These contrast obsessions are far from uncommon. We
have a case in the wards, a woman of sixty, who, every
time she enters a church, is assailed by erotic images,
which are caused by an occurrence that upset her very
much one day during a menstrual period.

We have had another woman, who suffered from erotic
and agonizing ideas whenever, in church, she found herself
looking at sacred images, chiefly the Way to the Cross
or the pictures of the tortures of the Saints.

These contrast obsessions correspond to a psychological
process, which Freud has brought out in connection with
the interpretation of dreams. The dream, says Freud,
often brings together contrary things and represents them
as a single object. In the cases that are of interest to us,

the conscience takes part in the conflict between these contrary elements. It is in this that there is the origin of a recrudescence of agony which becomes so intense as to drive these patients to suicide, especially when they imagine that mysterious forces are at the root of these states ; the two cases mentioned above thought they were demoniacal forces and were in despair about it.

The contrast obsessions, when they are accompanied by a permanent dissociation of the personality, end in insanity. The psychoneurotic become psychotic. We rediscover them at the beginning of the case-history of certain insane people, whose psychosis has begun by some such phenomena ; these insane are convinced that a foreign personality has taken possession of them and is driving them in the opposite direction to which their natural tendencies would lead them. Seglas has made a study of such cases under the title of the persecuted-possessed ; they are also the cases that show manifestations of the mental automatism of M. de Clérambault. We shall not stop to deal with such cases here ; that would be to digress from our subject.

The cases of obsession by contrast head the list of the emotive. Others are of this same morbid constitution, described by Dupré, which is characterized by exaggerated reflexes, rapidity and augmentation of response of the tendon reflexes, increase in the pupillary reflex, and cutaneous reflexes as well as increase in response of the vaso-motor reflexes.[1]

Another category of patient also comes under the heading of emotive psychoneurosis ; those cases who suffer from nightmares that recall the demonic oppression of the Middle Ages. Coelius Aurelianus has laid stress on the sensations these cases feel, a feeling of suffocation accompanied by marked anxiety and such conditions as the illusion that some spirit or devil is abusing their body.

Besides the association of contrary things, we find in

[1] E. Dupré, " Les déséquilibres constitutionnels du system nerveux," *Paris médical*, Jan., 1919.

these patients another association, which forms the very basis of Freud's doctrine, the association of anxiety and sexual emotion. Indeed it is Freud's teaching that anxiety is the result of the repression of the sexual tendencies.

The psychoanalysts have frequently found this association in such states as those of obsessions. These facts may be explained by the psychoanalytic mechanism and also by a physiological mechanism ; the centres of anxiety and the centres of the sexual life belong to the same vagal system, the former being bulbar, and the latter sacral. M. Laignel-Lavastine has on several occasions emphasized the relationship of these two groups of centres.

The patients, who suffer from oppressive nightmare, also suffer from digestive troubles, the commonest of which are air-swallowing and gaseous distension of the colon. We have found the presence of air-swallowing in every case in which the patient complained of anxiety dreams, and the feeling of an external presence which oppresses him and stops his respiration.

C. Aurelianus had already pointed out the importance of this point, and the interpreters of dreams had noted that a certain number of dreams depended, when they occurred in the first part of the night, on digestive troubles. Moreover, the disciples of Artemidorus of Ephesus had made the recommendation never to attempt the interpretation of dreams, that occurred in the first part of the night, for they might have been caused by the slow digestion of the heavy feasts of antiquity.

The contrast obsession, the nightmare oppression, appear as well-defined syndromes. But besides these there is a whole series of other depressive syndromes, in which the devil plays a rôle, either in his classical form, or in the form of evil forces. It is here that it is necessary to introduce the factor of imagination, which is of great importance in all these phenomena, for it is this that gives them the appearance in which they are presented. It then becomes a question of hysteria, a variety of psychoneurosis which has an imaginative basis.

The imagination thus produces suggestions of diverse origin; sometimes it is a question of beliefs directly inherited from the old Demonology with the additions which this has brought to orthodox religious belief; sometimes it is a question of more recent beliefs, either spiritualistic or theosophical. The forms of the manifestations in these two cases are variable.

We have studied the case of a woman, whose exalted imagination had been encouraged by the circle in which she lived, in a province of central France, in which one still finds quite a number of sorcerers. This woman seemed to mistake herself for one of the demoniacs of the Sabbaths of former times. We have seen her abandon herself to dances and contortions such as were formerly depicted in drawings of gatherings of sorcerers or in exorcismal ceremonies. Such attitudes formerly had been the cause of grouping all the demonopathies in the vast class of hysteria. Paul Richer, who had been Charcot's assistant, has illustrated his " Lectures at the Salpêtrière " with drawings of hysterical patients in their crises that recall the attitudes in the old engravings.[1]

In this patient the contortions disappeared on treatment by the method that M. Babinski still uses, persuasion aided by the electrical machine; and with them the attacks of possession disappeared also. This patient, during the time she was dancing, spoke in a strange voice, as if another person inhabited her body; she behaved as one possessed   Since then all these phenomena have given way to a state of ordinary hyper-emotivity.

These phenomena greatly interested me; they are very rare in this form, but they have been noted in other cases in an attenuated but very characteristic form. I refer to the trance of mediums.

If one studies these trances, one notes that they begin by a series of irregular respiratory movements; the

---

[1] Cf. *Bibliothèque diabolic de Bourneville* : Le Sabbat des Sorciers, François Fontaine, La Possession de Jeanne Ferry, Sœur Marie des Anges.

respiration rate instead of being 16 per minute, rises to 25 or 30, and sometimes more. There is also a proportionate tachycardia ; the pulse becomes more and more rapid and in the end the patient sweats profusely. It is beyond all doubt that the first irregular respiratory movements are voluntarily produced and in this is it a question of a form of simulation that is intended to liberate the powers of the unconscious ? In this patient simulation is less in evidence and it is our belief that we are dealing with a case of hysteria, since the treatment relieved not only the motor but also the intellectual phenomena, from the time when it was first applied. This treatment would have been without effect on the persecuted-possessed ; in this fact there is a diagnostic aid in differentiating between psychoneurosis and psychosis.

One finds in the emotive psychoneurosis as in hysteria, in a great number of cases, symptoms of asthenia, which may be either constitutional or acquired. Let me roughly summarize the symptoms of asthenia.

Asthenia is characterized by fatigability, resulting in difficulty in undertaking or sustaining effort. The patient is incapable of persevering in his efforts and, at the end of a very short time feels symptoms of fatigue. At this time there is added a second symptom having a very peculiar character ; irritability, which shows itself in two forms—anxiety or impatience.

Some constitutional asthenics have always been weak, the people for whom existence is a burden and for whom the contact with life is particularly painful. Here are some of the characteristics observed in a constitutionally asthenic woman, studied in the *Journal de psychologie*, of October, 1926, Marie von Mörl, who at times was a demoniacal mystic :

" Maria had never been well. At the age of five she spat up blood as the result of a stomach trouble, and in her ninth or tenth year she had a recurrence which again caused blood-spitting, oppression, and a constantly painful spot in the left side.

" She could not make long vocal prayers, but she prayed all the more interiorly and in contemplation. . . . Often, for hours at a time, she suffered considerably from melancholy, suspicious fear, anxiety, irritation, etc."

Marie von Mörl was a typical constitutional asthenic. She died at the age of fifty-five having passed her whole life in bed.

Other cases, who come under the category of acquired asthenia, have become run down as the result of grief or illness ; these griefs and illnesses inhibit the psychic control and are largely accountable for mediumistic phenomena and especially automatic writing. These mediumistic phenomena, which are made more pronounced by training and practice, are particularly dangerous because they offer illusion for the consolation of grief. The sensibility, become more subtle, guides the forces of an unconscious, that has been delivered into the hands of itself. This unconscious functions according to the laws, which one is beginning to appreciate in the so-called " hypnotic " states, which served as the basis of the first psychoanalytic studies. In the hypnotic state, as in the mediumistic trance or in the vision of seers,[1] the associations of ideas, instead of being guided by logic, are grouped together by affective ties, symbolic thought is general, and allusive play of words, and assonances all unite the elements of a thought, which is but half coherent, but which contains sometimes interesting intuitive fragments.

The constitutional or occasional asthenics seek ways that will liberate them from the feeling of their own weakness; from irritation, from anxiety, from impatience. They wish to escape from these painful impressions. They find these paths if they have been prepared for them by education or sometimes by their dispositions being hereditarily mystic. If this mysticism be not guided by higher controls, as St. Theresa considered essential, they

[1] Jean Vinchon, " Une mystique du Tyrol : Marie de Mörl," *Journal de Psychologie*, Oct., 1926.

fall into reveries and sensual ecstasies, to speak in the manner of the Carmelite founder. In these ecstasies, the instincts take the leading place and direct the interior life, especially at such times as evening, when work is done, when the distractions of everyday life give place to quieter hours, more removed from the world ; one witnesses then the opening of a thought which has been described by Bleuler—the " autist " thought that has lost its contact with the world, that characterizes the schizoid, a form of thought that evidences the dissociation of a subject turned back upon himself. Little by little he has become the prisoner of his own dream.

Right from the moment when the individual is caught by his own dream, he leads a dual life. This dual life is very curious. The letter, which my friend Maurice Garçon, and I have received some time back, depicts very well this double psychology.

It concerns a woman of forty-five, a widow. Here are several passages from it :

" I dream, or in other words I live a double life. Some years ago a priest of this part of the country, who made my acquaintance in a dream, said to me in a dream : ' She is possessed by the devil.' I vaguely knew the expression on the one hand, and on the other I knew that I dreamed. But I had never associated the two ideas. Since then I have tried to read and to make the acquaintance of people who were interested in my case, and you are the first who has answered me. . . .

" I live a dual existence, and how is that ? Sleeping the complete night, that is to say the full number of hours between going to bed and getting up, how is it that I have time to live complete with movement and action, another day between the day before and the following morning ? . . .

" Here is the scientific explanation that the devil has given me. . . .

" I don't speak of this before my children. . . .

" However, I am in control of my actions ; I live my

life more or less just as I want to ; in my good periods I am free."

This woman says that she hides her dream life from her children, and keeps it to herself. She lives two lives, one completely independent of the outside world, and the other adapted to the outside world. This doubling of the personality is characteristic of the schizoid. Grief, at the loss of her husband, had caused in this case the asthenia which induced the doubling of the personality. The schizoid may stop at this stage or may go on to such insane reveries, as are described by the Swiss alienists of Bleuler's school, as schizophrenia and by Chaslin as "folie discordante" ; the insanity then becomes the refuge of these people against the hypersensibility of their psyche.

Following the plan of these lectures, having demonstrated the appearance of the phenomena from the psychic aspect, we shall attempt to go deeper and see what one can find in these people from the organic point of view.

The *organic examination* of these cases, contrast obsessions, the emotive suffering from nightmare oppression, asthenics who are more or less schizoid, gives some interesting information.

One finds in the first categories the symptoms of the emotive constitution of Dupré, with, in the sympathetic field, the different types of unequilibrium of this system : vagotonia, hyper-ortho-sympathicotonia or amphotonia, that is to say the association of the first two types.

In these people epilepsy is not uncommon ; the ancient writers had already noted this fact ; tabes appeared to have had a part in one of our cases and proved that the primary real defects of sensibility had been interpreted as secondary.

Morphologically, the general appearance of these cases, of these women—for it is usually women who suffer from these conditions—often is that of the clinical picture described by M. Laignel-Lavastine in his lecture on hypotensive psychoneurosis.

From the endocrine viewpoint, the troubles observed are due to involvement of secretions of various glands, but chiefly of the ovary and the thyroid. It chiefly affects women about the menopause, which has a repercussion on the glands as have also worries, bereavements, widowhood, or the loss of a child, all of which rock the psyche, producing a train of circumstances which favours the creation of these compensating dreams. In this complex state the physical symptoms of anxiety are mixed with endocrine and neuro-psychiatric symptoms.

Among the organic affections that evolve parallel to these states, one must first mention digestive troubles ; they are almost as frequent in the demoniac psychoneuroses as in one psychosis, in which they are almost the rule—hypochondria. One finds also in these cases ptoses and, especially in those who suffer from nightmare oppression, there occurs gaseous distension of the colon, air-swallowing, delayed digestion, and a chronic coated state of the digestive tube. There is a close connection between the ordinary nightmare of the air-swallower and the nightmare found in our patients ; the initial sensation of respiratory suffocation is found in both. This is due to the diminution in amplitude of the inspirations, a diminution often favoured by the morphology of the patient. Many of them have a small thorax and a well developed abdomen, which gives the air-swallower the very characteristic appearance described by M. Leven. Goose-flesh also is common, the sensation of cold sometimes alternating with burning sensations, of which the victims of oppression complain very much and which is a feature of both ancient and modern stories of demoniacs. This particular phenomenon gives the subject the sensation of contact with the demon or with a materialized spirit.

Apart from these digestive troubles one often finds in these patients skin troubles, such as pruritus, urticaria, crops of acne, aggravation of latent eczema, isolated cutaneous troubles or such as are related to the digestive troubles. Such troubles have a bad effect on the patient and increase their discomfort ; they can be noted to occur chiefly in the periods of crisis.

There is another variety of trouble that is quite curious in that it had a considerable importance in the Middle Ages—the cheloïdes—which are of common occurrence in vagotonics. They were formerly taken to be marks of the demon on account of the changes in sensibility that is seen at their level.

With regards to general diseases, syphilis would not appear to play any important part. On the other hand, tuberculosis is extremely frequent, especially in the forms in which asthenia predominates. Our demoniac mystic of the Tyrol, Maria von Mörl, had a suspicious blood-stained sputum during the whole of her youth and the pious paintings, in which she is depicted, show her as a woman in a very feeble state, fatigued and always in bed, where she passed the greater part of her life.

The *evolution* of the demoniac psychoneuroses is often paroxysmal. It is rarely chronic, is only so in the insane ; in our cases, who are neuropaths, the attacks return, in more acute form, at certain times, under the influence of psychic or physical causes, while at other times there are periods of intermission.

The *prognosis* must depend on the clinical form of the psychoneurosis and the soil it is in.

The knowledge of the soil in which the condition has developed is here of first importance. It has been said that the soil in which mysticism can flourish is rare to-day. A very short enquiry in mystic or theosophic circles will suffice to show that it is more common than one would have supposed. The taste for the supernatural is still as widespread as ever, and if it does not satisfy itself in the established forms of religion, it appears on the least hesitation or doubt when facing the important problems of life. The fashionable fortune-teller of to-day numbers in his clientèle, politicians and financiers, who are otherwise known to be hard-headed and sceptic in their professional capacities.

The prognosis, then, varies according to the clinical form and the soil in which the condition is. The contrast obsessions have a grave prognosis ; they are almost all complicated by pathological doubt, as in the case of Séglas' young girl patient, and they end in such chronic conditions as chronic hallucinatory psychosis.

With M. Laignel-Lavastine, we have had under observation, at the St. Anne Hospital, a priest who suffered from contrast obsessions. These, which at the start had been only pure obsessions, soon came to have a demented character. While he said the Mass, a force took possession of him and prevented him from saying the words of the sacrament. He ended by saying these words with such violence that it caused a scandal and he was forced to perform his offices in a chapel apart. But the condition became of more and more frequent occurrence and one day he felt the devil take possession of him.

As a general rule, the prognosis of contrast obsessions is bad. On the other hand the nightmare oppression, if uncomplicated, is a benign syndrome. It disappears as soon as the air-swallowing is treated. The Church no longer includes it amongst the diabolic manifestations, a fact which at once allows one to show its true nature to patients.

The physical treatment is directed towards the obsessions and the asthenia. But in this one has to take account of the special character of these neuro-psychic syndromes, know the elements of diabolic mysticism, and enroll competent and reasonable religious help, for in many cases medicine alone will be insufficient and here, more than anywhere else, the physician should remain within the limits of his profession. Such patients have a distrust of him and it will be almost always necessary to bring a religious authority into the treatment.

Now that we have run over the general characteristics of the psychoneuroses of demoniac tint, we shall stop for a moment at a particular case, that will give us important evidence on the significance of the soil as a predisposing cause. The condition cropped up, predisposed to by heredity, after a life which scarcely seemed to have been favourable to the development of mystic tendencies, in fact the opposite. In the course of this observation we shall come across symptoms of different psychoneuroses which we have separated for the sake of descriptive purposes.

Notes on M.H.G. This is the case of a patient who had gone through a very terrible attack before being treated, first at the Salpêtrière and then in this service. He is fifty-seven years of age. He has suffered from the trouble under discussion for eighteen months. He is a photographic lithographer ; he worked at this occupation till 1922, at which time he had to give up his work. During a tragic outburst he attempted the life of his small son, after which he stabbed himself with a dagger. This took place in Brittany. He was arrested and taken to the Hospital at Quimper, and thereafter did six months of preventative prison. He was brought to trial and the jury unanimously acquitted him.

After this attack he explained : (1) That he was under the domination of something in himself, that a sort of auto-suggestion had ended by bringing him to this act ; (2) that he had had a revelation and that he attempted to take his child's life in order to deliver it from life and " in order that it might not turn out badly."

This is a clear-cut case of contrast obsession : He loved his child with very marked affective tendencies and at the same time felt himself driven towards homicidal tendencies.

Interrogation of the patient :

Q.—At the time of this happening, had you been hearing voices ?

A.—I haven't heard any voice, what I feel and what I felt is impossible to describe.

Q.—How do these manifestations appear ?

A.—I have seen no signs.

Q.—How do you react to these sensations ?

A.—I have not reacted. I have often tried to define what was going on within me. I couldn't.

Q.—Are there any special ideas that enter your mind ?

A.—I do nothing but reflect, and philosophize.

Q.—Are there any mental images that accompany those manifestations ?

A.—Yes, there are many, they come all the time, it's like a cinema.

Q.—Are these images very painful ?

A.—Generally very painful.

Q.—Consequently, there is an emotion of sensitiveness, of anguish, at the same time as the images, and all this repeats itself ?

A.—All the time. I should like to be free of it all.

Q.—The anguish is constant ?

A.—Yes, but the images vary.

Q.—Do they oppose each other ?

A.—Most of the time there is no continuity !

Q.—When you like a person very much, you sometimes have the idea of doing them harm ?

A.—Yes, I have contrary feelings. If I seek to console myself with happy thoughts, they soon become terrible.

(Here are two contradictory feelings for the same thought, which illustrate very well the continually contradictory tendencies of the affectivity of these cases, from which derives their contradictory conduct, affectionate or hostile.)

Q.—Have you been successful in freeing yourself from this ?

A.—No.

Q.—Are you tired, nervous ?

A.—Always ; there are times when I am quarrelsome and fight. (This is the irritability of the asthenic.)

Q.—These obsessions came on you little by little ?

A.—Yes, but not very long ago.

Q.—How did they begin ?

A —It's very hard to say. They were less frequent at
first. I had a first phenomenon, a sort of paralysis
of the right arm, I was afraid I might become
paralysed. Everything became progressively worse,
like a fog coming down.

Q.—When you had yielded to those acts, to which you
had felt driven, did you feel eased ?

A —Yes, I was very much easier, even extraordinarily so.

Q.—At that time you felt your arm swollen, and you had
a feeling of oppression of your heart ? Did you
tremble ?

A.—Yes, I had trembling of the right leg, and my heart
felt oppressed.

(Four years ago this man had had a period of relative
calm, after the first attack, which ended in the way
we know. Then came a second attack : the
patient thought he had syphilis. Incidentally he
had a history of a chancre.)

Q.—At the present time you again have ideas that chase
through your mind ?

A.—Yes, it hasn't stopped. I'm only quiet when I'm
asleep.

Q.—You have become more and more tired and apt to
be irritable, as in your first attack. But you haven't
dreamed and you have never heard voices ?

A.—No ; but I am always tired.

(This case is very different from the one who hears
voices, ordering him to do things he does not wish
to do, who is the victim of psycho-motor impulses.
Anguish in this case has become a marked feature,
he has the sensation of being a prisoner.)

A.—Indeed, I am not free to do what I want.

(This is extremely interesting, because we are here on
the threshold of a demoniac state. The patient
states : " It's as if someone prevented me from
doing what I want," but this remains in the state
of feeling without becoming objective ; there is no
force properly speaking that takes possession of

him. Nevertheless in his dreams he has representations of the devil.)

A.—I had that not in a dream, but when awake, during the day.

(These are facts such as one finds very commonly in stories of ancient sorcery.)

He has also the impression of water, drops of rain, that fall round him ; again this rain and these drops are found in tales of sorcery.

At this time the patient states that he does not dream at night.

Q.—Do you feel that someone has taken possession of your thoughts ?

A.—No, I am still master of my thoughts.

Q.—How did you know that there were evil thoughts in you ?

A.—I cannot explain what drove me, it was a sort of sensation. I was astonished that such a thought should follow me and I realized that this sensation did not really exist.

(His father had tendencies towards mysticism ; he himself was brought up in a very religious atmosphere, then several years ago he became quite irreligious ; at the present he has become religious again. In addition, he has had sensations of fright, the fear of becoming insane, of being lost.)

A.—I try to resist this fright, I watch myself, I force myself to take long walks.

He feels himself a prisoner, has the impression that he is gripped in his clothes as if he were tied up. He has diabolical visions, dreams of snakes, but he cannot tell his dreams, which he says he can't remember, and also he does not dream much.

From the organic aspect he suffers from hypertension, probably of luetic origin ; his blood pressure is 18/10 with the Pachon machine.[1]

From the neuro-vegetative point of view, one finds the

[1] See footnote on p. 44.

solar reflex distinctly positive, the oculo-cardiac reflex is nil; the manifestations are in the main of psychic origin. But an interesting point, that has a relationship to the work of M. Laignel-Lavastine and Cornelius in this service, is that the pH is distinctly on the alkaline side, at 7, 2.

With regard to the other symptoms, if we summarize the notes on this case, we see produced the complex clinical picture of these cases of asthenia with contrast obsessions, predisposed to by heredity and favoured by the organic conditions present, such as hypertension, relative hepatic insufficiency (pH alkaline) and syphilis. The knowledge of the morbid character of these phenomena is sufficient in itself to differentiate a case of this sort from the mystic or demoniac insane.

We started with facts which appeared to the uninformed to be foreign to medicine. In submitting these facts to the rules of clinical observation and medical criticism,[1] we have uncovered a part of their mystery and have grouped them with these psychoneuroses with which you are now acquainted. We have succeeded sometimes in curing, sometimes in relieving these cases, who are too often the victims of empirical treatment. The treatment, in showing us the nature of the diseases and in improving the conditions of the sufferers, brings us the best conclusion of this study essay of the demoniac psychoneuroses.

[1] Maurice Garcon et Jean Vinchon, " Le Diable," in *Documents bleus*, 1926.

VII

THE SYMPATHETIC AND ENDOCRINE REACTIONS IN THE PSYCHONEUROTIC

BEFORE taking up with you the sympathetic and endocrine reactions in the psychoneurotics, I want to remind you that, in the concentric method of diagnosis of the psychoneurotic, there is the need to investigate in succession the psychic zone, neurological zone, endocrine zone, the visceral zone, and last the morbific kernel. I have seen with pleasure that M. Achard, in his opening lecture to his class at the Beaujon Hospital, has demonstrated a method which corresponds to what I have called the diagnosis in depth,[1] and it is very true that there is only one way of getting to the bottom of the patients' conditions and making a complete diagnosis.

In demonstration of this very complex question, I shall first review the study of the schema ; I shall consider the methods of examining the nervous and endocrine zones by several concrete examples ; I shall show you how one may apply the important theoretical facts and I shall give you some aspects of the conception of the order of sympathetic, endocrine and psychic symptoms.

Examination of the nervous zone.—I have told you that it was necessary to investigate two aspects : the *neurological aspect of relationship* and the *sympathetic aspect*.

The methods of investigation of the aspect of relationship are quite classical. It is the study of the semeiology of all the reflexes and of all the modifications of sensibility that one ordinarily looks for in sensory-motor neurology, and there is not a better way than that of M. Babinski, which consists in seeing *whether there is*

[1] Achard, *Presse médicale*, 1927.

present or not physical signs of an organic lesion affection of the nervous system. This is the main point, the Ariadne's thread.

Alongside this group—physical signs of organic lesion affection of the nervous system—there is the possibility of finding a certain number of modifications, which, while they do not allow one to affirm the presence of an organic lesion, nevertheless come under what I have called the *dynamic nervous organic semeiology*, and Babinski and Froment have shown that these disturbances, which they have called the *physiopathic syndromes*, if they are not the expression of an organic lesional change, still are neither the simple resultant of a process of purely psychic origin. This is an extremely important group from the point of view of what we are considering now, for the analysis of the physiopathic phenomena shows that there is a sympathetic factor in their determinism.

The study of this neurological aspect of relationship enables one to take into account very precisely everything which results from both the *organic lesional semeiology* and the *organic dynamic semeiology*.

Study of the sympathetic aspect.—The study of the sympathetic aspect could lead me very far indeed and take up several lectures, so I shall refer you to the researches I have already done and particularly to the very complete semeiological analysis which I have given not in my *Sympathetic Pathology*,[1] but in an article on the Sympathetic Chain, which has appeared in fascicle 36 of the *Traité de Médicine et Thérapeutiqul* of Gilbert and Carnot.[2] You will find in this, as also in the report of my friend André Thomas,[3] made at the last annual neurological congress, an enumeration of all the sympathetic reflexes that should be investigated in the study of disturbances of this system.

But before making this enumeration, a general remark

[1] Laignel-Lavastine, *Pathologie du sympathique*, In. 8, Alcan, 1924.
[2] Laignel-Lavastine, *Pathologie du nerf grand sympathique*, Baillière, 1924.
[3] André Thomas, *Revue neurologique*, Masson, 1926.

is necessary : it is that the responses to the elicitation of sympathetic reflexes are only valid for the territory which has been stimulated and for the territory on which depends the reflex which is concerned in the response. In short, as Professor Bar has rightly shown, one must not believe that it is sufficient to stimulate any level of the sympathetic system to form an opinion of the degrees of excitability of its different fields. What is true for the rest of the cerebro-spinal system is true for the sympathetic. Although there is a great diffusion of sympathetic reflexes, there are territorial arrangements loosely enough connected together, and one must have this idea well in mind in order to understand the results, which, at the first glance, might appear to be contradictory.

Besides this, in the elicitation of sympathetic reflexes, as in the case of the tendon reflexes of the cerebro-spinal system, the important law of asymmetries is dominant, especially in lesional sympathetic semeiology. This asymmetry of reflexes of one side in comparison to the other must immediately make one think of the existence of a local lesion.

I now pass to the enumeration of the different reflexes which should be investigated in coming to a conclusion as to the state of the sympathetic system of any psychoneurotic.

1. In the first place, the *vaso-motor cutaneous reflexes.*— The skin is, indeed, a wonderful field from the point of view of the ease with which variations in vaso-motor state can be observed.

The *meningitic streak*, classical from the time of Trousseau, is characteristic of vaso-dilatation, while, when vaso-constriction follows vaso-dilatation, the *white streak* of Vulpian is got. The thyroidean *red mark*, studied by Marañon, is produced by friction over the anterior aspect of the thyroid. Sergent's *white line*, misnamed " suprarenal," does not always coincide with adrenal insufficiency; it can be produced in the moment after death, before idiomuscular excitability has disappeared from the skin, when the big neurones are already dead ; this fact shows that it depends on idio-muscular excitability.

In addition, the *white streak*, which I described with Hallion, gives an idea of the activity of the local circulation, and gives valuable results when compared with the curves got with the Pachon oscillometer. Further, the results got with the Vaquez-Laubry apparatus permits of numerous things being noted. Here is one : When one takes the arterial blood-pressure with this apparatus, by the auscultatory method, one first hears a strong beat, which, as one lets out the pressure, is replaced by a particular *humming*, which lasts a certain time, and which disappears before the end of the sound coinciding with the diastolic pressure ; I believe that the strength of this humming-vibration, in relationship to the systolic and diastolic figures got with the Vaquez-Laubry machine, may be of use in certain forms of sympathetic disturbance.

The plethysmographic method with the Hallion and Conte apparatus measures the vaso-motor variations produced by the application of ice, according to the Josué method, by the hot bath test of Babinski and Heitz and by hydrotherapy. Capillaroscopy, epidermolyscopy, the methodical scratching or, better, graduated epidermolysis, and lastly the intradermal reaction throw light in part on the local cutaneous nervous situation.

2. After the analysis of the cutaneous vaso-motor reflexes comes the study of the *cutaneous thermal reactions*. *Anisothermy* has an important place in sympathetic semeiology. Babinski has shown the relative frequency of anisothermy in the syndromes of pontine lesions.

The most important sympathetic reflex, from the point of view of precise localization of sympathetic lesions, is the *Pilo-Motor reflex*, which has been admirably studied in a monograph of André Thomas. Then comes the *Sudatory reflexes*, which pharmaco-dynamically are dependent on the vagal system, but anatomically, on the orthosympathetic.

Then, the various *pharmaco-dynamic reflexes*, that are

produced by the subcutaneous injection of 1 cc. of 1 in 1,000 adrenalin, by subcutaneous injection of 1 cgm. of pilocarpine, or 1 milligm. of eserine, or 1 milligm. of the neutral sulphate of atropine, or lastly by the inhalation of v minims of amyl nitrite.

3. From the pharmacological reflexes, produced by chemical substances, we pass to the consideration of *Biological tests*, such as, the injection of hypophyseal substance as in Claude and Porak's method, injections of thyroid substance as in Parisot's method, and the injection of insulin. Then we come to the most important of all the sympathetic reflexes, the *Oculo-Cardiac Reflex*.

Many objections have been raised to this reflex, because it may by its method of use lead to many errors, but by knowing how to interpret its results it becomes of extreme importance, to the extent that I would say that *the oculo-cardiac reflex is to sympathology what the knee-jerk is to sensory-motor neurology*. Many of the *forms of visceral sympathico-vagal reflexes* are only derivatives of the oculo-cardiac reflex.

Amongst the most interesting reflexes let us also note the *Solar reflex*, by means of which we estimate the excitability of the orthosympathetic ; the *Naso-facial reflex*, which has been studied by my friend Paul-Emile Weil and which gives information on the vegetative system of the face. One of my pupils, M. Louge, has shown the importance of the *Palato-cardiac reflex*, which gives one information on the sympathetic or the vagus according to the way in which one tickles the soft palate.

The *digestive-haemoclasis test*, discovered by M. Widal, who originally considered it as furnishing information on liver function, has been taken up again by several authorities and found susceptible of having a significance in many cases, from the semeiological point of view.

To carry out this test, the patient is given 200 grms. of milk in the fasting state. Studies are thereafter made of the changes that occur in the sympathetic field, in the vagus field, and in the blood from the viewpoint of white cell count, colour index, its H-ion concentration, refracto-metric index, and surface tension.

Proceeding to reflexes of greater and greater complexity, I come to the study of the basal metabolism, which is of great importance in clinical sympathetic pathology, for it is actually the best way we have of informing ourselves of the state of activity of the Thyroid gland, the gland of emotion which plays such a large part in the sym-pathetic nervous system.

The basal metabolism, which is the opposite of the maximal metabolism, is the energy, expressed in calories (that is to say the amount of heat required to raise a litre of water one degree Centigrade), expended per hour per square metre of body surface by an individual who is in a state of complete rest, who has fasted for about 14 hours and who is placed in an average atmosphere of 16 deg. (Cent.), and covered so as not to react to cold or heat in his surroundings. This basal metabolism is increased in hyperthyroidism, and diminished in thyroid insufficiency. In actual practice, instead of making the expression in calories, it is usually more simply stated as a percentage of increase or decrease above or below a predicted stan-dard, based on age, weight, sex, etc.

The *pupillary reflex* gives information on changes in the cerebro-spinal and sympathetic systems. Schiff's reaction consists in dilatation of the pupil by pain. Tournay's reaction is dilatation occurring in the outwards deviated eye when the eyes are moved laterally. Mydriasis by cocaine or adrenalin occurs by stimulation of the sympathetic as does the mydriasis by atropine or the marked contraction of the pupil by pilocarpine.

An exaggerated naso-labial reflex response indicates hyperexcitability of the vagus.

It is perhaps true that modifications in the tendon reflexes allow us to make inductions of the same sort, but this is a question that has still to be studied.

When one has made this series of examinations, one brings together all the changes furnished by the study of these reflexes, and one groups them in two categories according to whether or not they correspond with the cases of lesional semeiology.   If there is asymmetry of reflex permitting of localization at a precise point, one says that there is a local lesion of the sympathetic.   This is a diagnosis of a local sympathetic syndrome.

On the contrary the variations, which are neither asymmetrical nor localized, but more or less diffuse, derive from a degree of excitability of the whole system, so that one places them in the group of dynamic sympathetic semeiology.

Having reviewed the possible manifestations in the nervous zone, let us now study the *endocrine zone.*

Here, again, there are two aspects to be considered, the *morphological aspect* and the *humoral aspect.*

Charcot, very justly, gave a very bad mark at clinical examinations to students who rushed at the patient without studying him in his general aspect.   In semeiology it is always important to take a general view, just like a painter or sculptor who wants to give a true rendering of his model.

Here are some cases that will serve me as examples :

1st *Case.*—Mme. Lune is a patient who has periods of depression.   From the morphological point of view her outstanding feature is her face, which shows a tendency almost exactly to describe a circle, and also some adiposity ;   she weighs 66 kilos. and is 152 cms. in height. She has a yellowish complexion, is somewhat swollen in appearance ;   her hands are large.   She is the hypothyroid type with diminished basal metabolism, and this thyroid insufficiency plays a part in her periods of depression.

2nd *Case.*—Mlle. Sylphide is a young girl who came to see us for a " grippe " ;   I wanted you to see her on account of her special morphology ;   she has good health, but she is extremely tall, 173 cms., and she weighs 52 kilos.   She is of the *longiform* type with legs like a stork.   Her length from the umbilicus to the vertex is much less than that from the umbilicus to the feet.   Radiography shows nothing abnormal. Sylphide has simply a series of minor ailments which shows that there are "false notes in her endocrine concert."

But it is not enough to study only the adiposity and the structure, one must take into account the variations in the skin from the point of view of pigmentation and hair distribution. You are aware of the importance, semeiologically, of the development of the hair, its scantiness in certain myxoedematous states, or its overgrowth, hypertrichosis, with a masculine disposition, that is got in the gynandroid.

Humoral aspect.—To complete the study of the endocrine zone, one must not be content with the morphology alone, a precise analysis of the modifications that are to be found in the body fluids is also necessary, to find if there is present a hyperadrenalinæmia, a hyper or hypoinsulinæmia, changes in blood sugar level, blood cholesterin and blood calcium, for the calcium metabolism plays an important part in endocrine disturbances, a diminution in calcium appearing to be parallel with a hyperexcitability of the vagus.

The variations in *hydrogen-ion concentration* must be studied. You are aware of the importance that has become attached to the pH that is the hydrogen-ion concentration, in the physico-chemical studies of the body fluids. The pH, whose theoretical basis is very complex, is a very simple investigation by the colorimetric method of Guillaumin. It has not got the precision of the electrometric method which M. Vincent worked out in the laboratory of M. Desgrez, but it is in the ordinary way of great use.

From the point of view which interests us, one must know that the hydrogen-ion concentration is normally expressed by figures, which run from about 5,8 to 6,6 and which gives with the Guillaumin reagent[1] a yellow

---

[1] Laignel-Lavastine et Cornelius, " Le pH urinaire et le titrage des acides organiques dans l'urine chez les anxieux et les déprimés,' Société de Biologie, Oct. 18, 1924, p. 872.

coloration, a slightly orange colour, or a colour that has a faint tinge of green in it.

When, however, the pH tends to rise considerably as in cases of *acidosis*, the figures are very low, beneath 5 and may go as low as 4.

When the tendency is towards *alkalosis* there is a marked diminution in the pH, the figures touch 7 and over, with an emerald green coloration ; this is the expression of an anxiety state. This very definite observation of a pH of over 7 characterized by an emerald green colour, coincides with an alkalosis. I have observed it very often in anxiety states, so much so that with M. Cornelius I was able to say that there was an anxiety associated with an increased urinary pH and that one could describe it as an " alkaline neurosis."

Having studied the morphological and humoral aspects of the patients, one can make an analysis of the endocrine troubles and distinguish the part played by the thyroid, parathyroid, ovary, pancreas, etc., in the disturbances under observation. I do not wish to go into detail and I shall simply give the facts, taking a few concrete examples of the application of the method that I have very rapidly shown you.

Let us take, for example, the pure case of " doubt," who, taking up a bundle of linen to put it in her apron, " cannot resist this force which compels her to look around several times on the ground to see if she has not left any, although she knows very well that she hasn't." I refer to the case of Mme. Thomas. This patient has an oculo-cardiac reflex which is considerably increased. Thus before applying ocular pressure, her pulse is 25 beats to the quarter-minute, and on compression the rate is only 13 ; there is thus a diminution of from 100 per minute to 52 beats per minute. On the other hand, epigastric compression gives a very poorly marked solar reflex. Thus this patient corresponds to a type, that we see frequently, of somewhat anxious doubt, with pure vagotonia, that is to say with the oculo-cardiac reflex considerably increased, while the other sympathetic manifestations are on the contrary normal. This is what I call *type* 1. Her urinary pH is materially normal ; it is 6.2. The interesting point is that Mme. Thomas' mother was also a sufferer from anxious doubt, so that one may ask oneself if the inherited doubt does not derive from a local hyperexcitability of the vagus and is not unconnected with a special anatomical disposition of the vagal nuclei and particularly the dorsal nucleus of the vagus.

We undoubtedly gain in being able to re-express a psychic clinical picture in the terms of the physiological formula of exaggeration of the oculo-cardiac reflex, which suggests the possibility of a constitutional anomaly of a very definite part of the brain stem, namely, one of the nuclei of origin of the pneumogastric nerve.

Examples of different types of modification of the oculo-cardiac reflex in their relationship to changes in the solar reflex.

Eppinger and Hess had thought from their early work that one could establish a relationship of inverse proportion between the excitability of the vagus and the excitability of the orthosympathetic. Now this theory does not fit what is generally actually found. Indeed, if one examines a large number of cases, as M. Largeau did in my service, from the point of view of the relationships between the oculo-cardiac reflex and the solar reflex, one can group them into four types :

First, there is what I call *type* 1, because it is the most frequent. It is characterized by *pure vagotonia* or almost so ; I have shown you one example in Mme. Thomas, the case of doubt, and here is another that I am going to show you.

3rd Case.—Here is Robert, a *myxoedematous dwarf*. He was admitted here with a temperature of 35.5 Cent., and under the influence of opotherapy and specific treatment—for he is a hereditary syphilitic—he has rapidly improved ; to-day he is able to work in the laboratory, but he still has a basal metabolism of —25 per cent., indicating

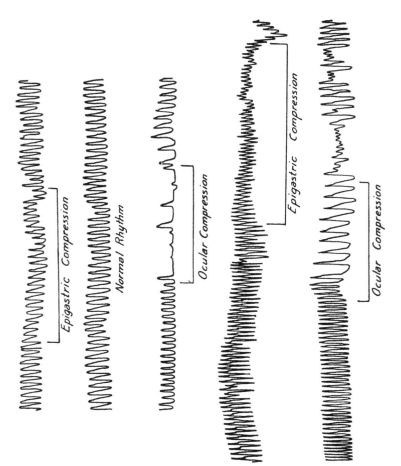

FIG. IV.—TYPE I. PURE VAGOTONIA.

that he still has a marked degree of thyroid insufficiency, and it is interesting to note that this insufficiency is accompanied by a considerable over-activity of his oculo-cardiac reflex, the pulse rate falling from 60 to 20 per minute, while there is scarcely any exaggeration of the solar reflex.

Type 1, then, is characterized by marked exaggeration of the oculo-cardiac reflex and absence or almost so of the solar reflex response.

Type 2 is the opposite type to this. The oculo-cardiac reflex is zero and the solar reflex is very exaggerated. There are cases where this exaggeration would appear to be due to anatomical factors.

Here, for example, is a woman who has an enormous gastric ptosis, causing dragging on the solar plexus and producing a marked exaggeration of the solar reflex ; ocular compression, on the other hand, causes no slowing of the pulse rate, whereas epigastric compression does effect a very great diminution in the rate. This is an example of *hyper-ortho-sympathicotonia*.[1]

Type 3 is the very common ; in it is found *exaggeration of both oculo-cardiac and solar reflexes*. There are, however, sub-varieties to be distinguished in this type 3.

There may be either—as you will see in an article I published on " Hygiene of patients with sympathetic irritability "[2]—an exaggeration of both oculo-cardiac and solar reflexes ; or the exaggeration may chiefly affect either the oculo-cardiac or the solar reflex.

Here are tracings, from a case of " scrupulous " psychasthenia, who has such an exaggeration of the solar reflex that he almost falls down in syncope on epigastric compression.

In another case the inverse is found, ocular compression produces almost disappearance of the radial pulse, while the solar reflex is much less affected.

---

[1] See footnote on p. 21.
[2] Laignel-Lavastine, " L'hygiène des irritables du sympathique," *Revue scientifique*, 1926, No. 1, p. 1, 8.

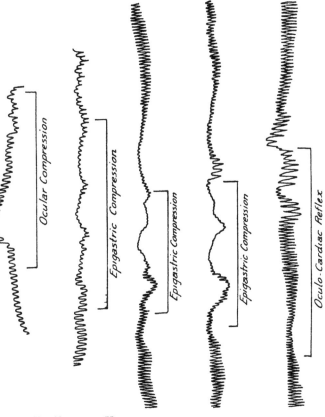

FIG. V.—TYPE 2. HYPERORTHOSYMPATHICOTONIA.

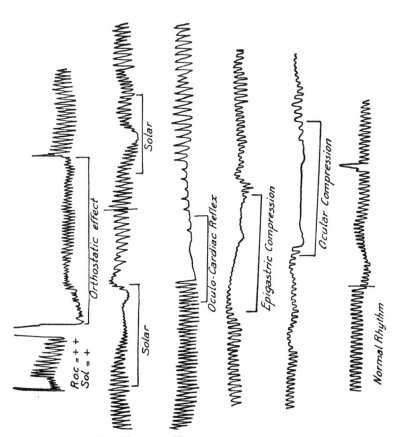

FIG. VI.—TYPE 3. HYPERHOLOSYMPATHICOTONIA.

Type 4 is characterized by a diminution in all the reflexes. This is very rare. You remember that here is a question of a general rule on which I laid stress at the beginning of this course of lectures ; if sensory-motor semeiology finds its best diagnostic indication in the phenomena of deficiency, the contrary is true in sympathetic semeiology which must receive its chief directions from manifestations of irritability, and the reason for this is that, in the sensory-motor system, the localizations of affections are extremely precise because one can easily establish in the brain stem the course of reflexes, whether centripetal or centrifugal. But in the sympathetic system, which is a system of relays formed of neurones with collateral and bifurcating branches, there is a very much greater diffusion of reflexes. Nevertheless type 4 is sometimes seen and here is an example.

This is the case of a woman, run down in health, with cephalalgy, who shows a normal solar reflex as well as an almost normal oculo-cardiac reflex. This leads me to say a word on the *normal limits* of these reflexes.

Considering the multiplicity of causes that produce variations in sympathetic excitability, one must not be rash in considering abnormal a patient who has a reflex more or less strong or more or less weak ; it is difficult to quote figures in this. It is a question for interpretation, all the more since there is an hourly curve of these reflexes. One knows that, other things being equal, vagus excitability is greater in the morning and in the fasting state, and that the excitability of the ortho-sympathetic is greater in the evening and after a meal. Also the physiological variations of these excitabilities has a relationship to the periodic variations of certain internal secretions, and so we come to the question of the relationships between the variations of sympathetic excitability and endocrine activity.

4th Case.—This is the case of Mme. Hotel. She is a young woman who states that, at about the age of fifteen,

L

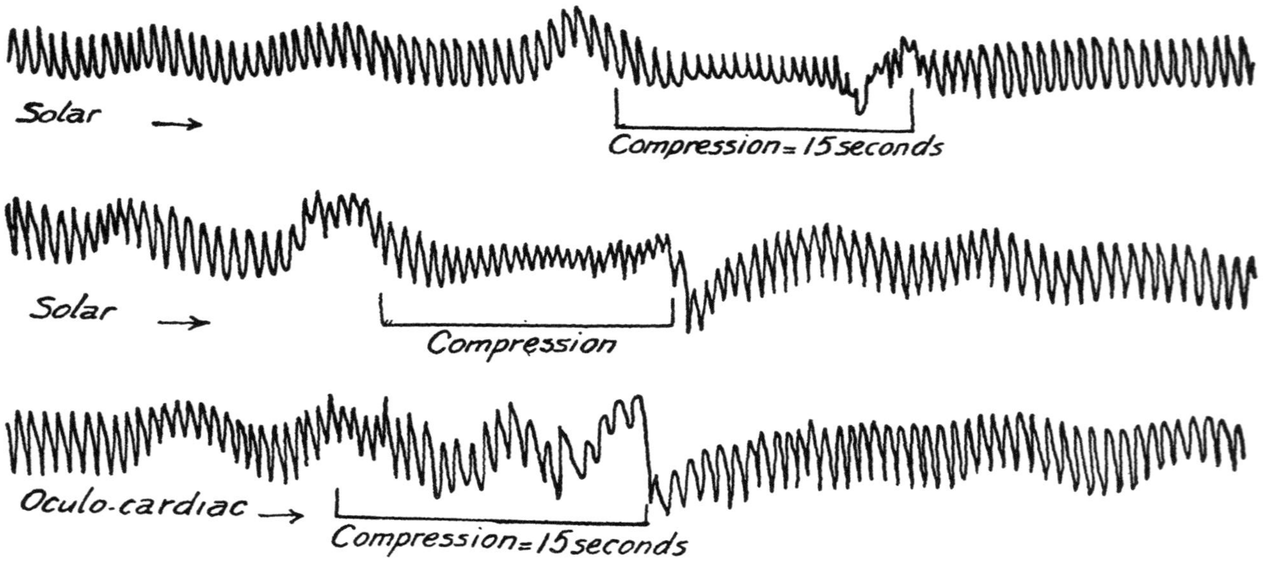

Solar →

Compression = 15 seconds

Solar →

Compression

Oculo-cardiac →

Compression = 15 seconds

FIG. VII.—TYPE 4. HYPOHOLOSYMPATHICOTONIA.

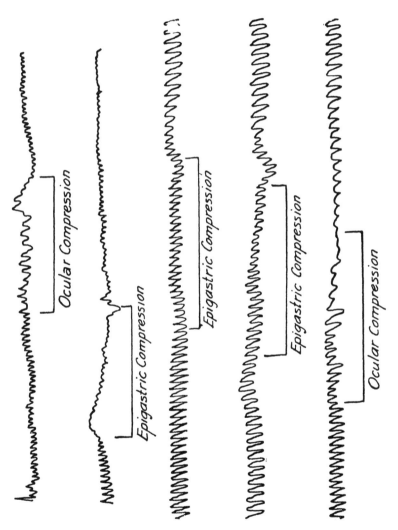

FIG. VIII. REACTION MARGIN IN NORMAL SYMPATHETIC.

she found herself in a lonely spot, near the fortifications, when all of a sudden she felt a strange empty feeling in her head. She felt as if she no longer existed, as if, she says, another person were in her. This lasted about half a minute, but, she says, the fear remained that " it might come on again," and because of this fear it certainly did so. Mme. Hotel now says that it is impossible for her to go into the woods alone, or to any other lonely place, without being accompanied, because she always has the fear that this horrible sensation will come back, " this emptiness in the brain, this cerebral anguish."

These phenomena appeared in this patient at puberty ; she has had very definite disturbance of the personality of the type of depersonalization, so well studied by Hesnard in his thesis, which seem to approximate the phenomena of *psycholepsy.* The individual suffers a diminution of his psychic make up, due to a diminution in psychological tension. This patient has retained from these phenomena a state of anxiety, and the point which interests us is that these anxiety manifestations, which persist, are superimposed on a very definite hyperthyroid foundation. One finds this in many of these cases, for the relationship between sympathetic disturbances and disturbance of thyroid function play an important part in these questions, and in this lies a separate aspect of the psychoneurotic pathology, which I shall discuss with you, in a future lecture, showing you a patient who, in a way, serves as an example of this.

Granted the analysis, which we have made of the neurological and endocrine zones, it is now worth while seeing how one can *arrange in order* these *sympathetic, psychic,* and *endocrine* disturbances.

To study them one must consider them in three different groups, because the best way of solving the difficulty is to divide it into as many subdivisions as it permits, according to the Cartesian principle.

I.—PSYCHO-SYMPATHETIC RELATIONS

I shall take four examples in relation to the four main varieties of the psychoneuroses : *hysteria, neurasthenia, psychasthenia,* and *emotive psychoneuroses.*

(*a*) Let us first consider *hysteria.* We had, six months ago, in this service, in the Brouardel ward, a young girl who was admitted with quite a remarkable hysterical hemi-anæsthesia of the left side. The first thought that came to one, according to Babinski's teaching, was that the hysterical hemi-anæsthesia had been caused by the suggestion of a doctor who must have said to the patient : " Do you feel less on one side than on the other ? " instead of " I am going to touch you and you will tell me what you feel." But on examining this girl more thoroughly, one noted that there was present a *vaso-motor asymmetry,* and that on the left side Vulpian's streak was white, while, on the right, the reaction was red.

This vaso-motor asymmetry appeared to me to be the cause of the suggestion of hemi-anæsthesia on the left side, and that by a process which was not medical hetero-suggestion. Indeed, it was Claude Bernard who first noted that there existed variations in sensibility related to sympathetic modifications, not in that the sympathetic fibres were conductors of tactile sensibility, but because section of the sympathetic, causing peripheral dilatation bathes the tactile corpuscles with a more generous and more easily renewed blood supply, in such a way that their sensibility threshold is lowered.

This observation has been repeated by my friend Tournay and, when one looks carefully, there is observable a variation in the threshold of tactile sensibility related to sympathetic changes. So here is an example, in which one is able to allocate to a regional variation in the sympathetic a hysterical auto-suggested hemi-anæsthesia.

(*b*) *Neurasthenia.*—The neurasthenic, we have said, are those who have periods of depression. From the point of view of their relationship to the sympathetic, they must be divided into two groups, according to whether one is dealing with a hypertensive or hypotensive neurasthenic.

There are *hypertensive cases* who owe their condition mainly to renal sclerosis, which produces a secondary hypertension. But others have a diminution in the height of the oscillations in the Pachon oscillometer due to a vaso-constriction factor, which plays a part in hypertension, and that one can diminish by the exhibition of amyl nitrite and benzyl benzoate.

As a rule the part played by the sympathetic is more clearly defined in the *hypotensive*. Indeed many hypotensive are so through adrenal insufficiency, as is also indicated by the diminution in both muscular and vascular tone.

(c) *Psychasthenia.*—In this connection let me recall to you our example of the case of " pure doubt " associated with a state of pure vagotonia.

Other cases are more complex, such as the *claustrophobes*, who have a fear of shut-in places. This is a type of marked vagotonia. Experimentally, Carnot has shown that an increase in carbonic acid in the organism stimulates the digestive part of the vagus, so that one might account for a fear of enclosed places in vagotonics by an exaggerated oxygen hunger, this uncomfortable condition arising from a rise in carbonic acid.

(d) *Emotive psychoneurosis.*—These very emotive people have a remarkable lability of the sympathetic and a considerable instability of their reactions. They show sometimes waves of heat, sometimes constrictive manifestations ; they are the people I have called *vaso-motor ataxics.*[1] This lability would often appear to be related to their adrenal reactions, particularly to adrenin discharge in relation to sympathetic changes. This is a point on which Cannon has laid much stress. He showed that in animals, particularly the dog, fear and rage were associated with a discharge of adrenin into the blood, and thus

[1] Laignel-Lavastine, *Leçons sur l'anatomie médicale des glandes endocrines,* Laennec, 1906.

in the emotive psychoneurotics one can show variations in blood adrenin, which would seem to be connected with psychosympathetic conduction.

And why, under the influence of emotions, do variations in blood adrenin so easily occur ? Because the adrenals are innervated by the Lesser Splanchnic nerves, which, like the Great Splanchnic, have this remarkable anatomical arrangement : their fibres arise in the lateral chain of the orthosympathetic and pass through the sympathetic ganglia without forming synapses there. Consequently the splanchnic system is, one might say, to the ortho-sympathetic almost what the vagal system is to the collective vegetative system. It is much more organized ; it is more intimately in touch with the synthesis of the individual and it is, in a way, a government already very centralized in comparison with the rest of the sym-pathetic, which one might consider as a federal govern-ment.

II.—THE RELATIONSHIP BETWEEN THE SYMPATHETIC AND THE ENDOCRINE GLANDS, AND ESPECIALLY BETWEEN THE THYROID AND THE SYMPATHETIC.

The sympathico-endocrine inter-relationships are com-plex and numerous, but I must limit myself to a field that is somewhat better known than the others, the field of reactions between the sympathetic and the thyroid. Even those are very complex. To limit ourselves, let us take, for example, the *relationship between the oculo-cardiac reflex and the state of thyroid function.*

I have shown you how frequent is the formula, oculo-cardiac reflex very exaggerated, solar reflex nil. In particular we have observed this in its typical manner in Robert, the hereditary syphilitic myxoedematous dwarf. We see the same thing in Jeanne, the marked hyper-emotive case, who has had symptoms of exophthalmic goitre, for which she was operated on by M. Sébileau.

Here are two cases in which the lesions are different, but who have the same sympathetic formula.

Let us further limit the question and take two cases of Basedow's disease, one that I have had in this service, who has had subcapsular thyroidectomy done, and who, in spite of this operation, still has a considerable degree of exophthalmos persisting, so much so that one was forced to have suture of the eyelids performed. In the second case also, the exophthalmos persisted in spite of operation.

Here, then, are two cases of Basedow's disease, in whom surgery had diminished the thyroid hyperfunction, but was without effect on the exophthalmos. From this it is evident that in these cases the syndrome of Basedow was not due entirely to a thyroid mechanism and that there was present a relatively independent sympathetic factor.

On the other hand, I have had, here, at consultation, a Roumanian physician, of whom I have already spoken to you, who was suffering from a very severe Basedow, characterized by a goitre and an extraordinary degree of exophthalmos and tachycardia. An operation had a remarkable effect on the tachycardia, but none on the exophthalmos, which also necessitated suture of the eyelids. I then advised him to have a resection of the cervical sympathetic performed. He refused this at first, but later decided to have it done ; he came to see me last month with a considerable amelioration in the exophthalmos.

This shows the complexity even of the symptoms in Basedow's syndrome and justifies the conception of my colleague and friend, Prof. Marcel Labbé, whose opinion is that there is an association of two pathogenic factors which do not completely react one on the other.

In the Basedow syndrome there is on the one hand disturbance of thyroid function, and on the other sympathetic disturbances, which may vary relatively with some independence.

Consequently, when faced with these manifestations, which are partly endocrine and partly sympathetic, one must not want immediately to establish an order relationship of causality, for this may be from the sympathetic to the endocrine gland, or from the gland to the sympathetic, but there is the possibility of the manifestations being parallel, deriving from an ulterior cause, like two branches that spring from the same trunk.

Psycho-sympathico-endocrine relationships. This field is still wider and more complex, since there is the added factor, the psychic factor.

To limit myself, I shall take in this factor, not a syndrome, but simply in a way what is a type reaction, the " anxious " type.

Anxiety is a complex, composed, from the psychic viewpoint, of insecurity, doubt and irresolution ; from the physiological point of view of vago-sympathetic disturbances varying with the intensity of the anxiety.

When the anxiety is slight, there is chiefly vagal excitability ; consequently the manifestations are characterized by a slowing of the pulse, occasional nausea, constipation and usually pallor.

If, on the other hand, the process is a prolonged one, from the fact of the law of diffusion of reflexes, the disturbances extend to the whole sympathetic system, and an orthosympathetic factor becomes added to the vagal factor.   Tachycardia is present, and there is some degree of dilatation of the pupil, tremor, redness of the face, and so one comes to the very markedly anxious type, in which is found a general hyperexcitation of the whole vago-sympathetic system, with a considerable concurrent motor agitation.

In this state of anxiety it becomes of importance to analyse the factors composing it, and with this object such an examination must be made as will enable one to decide whether one is dealing with one of the three following great varieties of anxiety : the *organic lesional* variety, the *psychogenetic* variety, or the *physiogenetic variety.*

The *organic lesional variety* undoubtedly exists ; there

are cases who owe their anxiety to a lesion, and with my friend Vigouroux I formerly cut sections, from old cases of melancholic anxiety with Cotard's syndrome, and found in the bulb, at the level of the dorsal nucleus of the vagus, an absolutely abnormal pigmentation. This, then, is the first form : *Organic lesional anxiety.*

But it is my belief that there exists not only an organic lesional anxiety ; there may occur an organic anxiety *due to anatomical anomaly.* You are all familiar with naevi, these skin stains or birthmarks. They are due to a cutaneous malformation, and sometimes they are the site of disturbances of sympathetic reaction indicating beyond all doubt the existence of an anomaly. Thus I once saw, at the St. Anne Hospital, a young girl who had a radiciform naevus corresponding to the lower cervical nerve roots. In the field of this naevus one could make out very definitely the absence of the pilo-motor reflex and also exaggeration of the white streak (of Vulpian) on local excitation, and, on the contrary, also manifestations of vaso-dilatation.

This contradiction was easily explained, it was my opinion that the condition was due to an absence of certain sympathetic cells in the left tractus intermedio-lateralis in the lower part of the cervical cord. This sympathetic syndrome was thus due to a developmental defect. I see no reason why one should not admit the possibility of a similar cause of manifestations which, instead of being organo-sympathetic, are psycho-sympathetic. And the female anxiety case, whom I showed you the other day, in whom the condition is hereditary, perhaps is so from an anomaly of some limited part of the dorsal nucleus of her vagus. A clinical argument in favour of this conception is the frequency of vagotonia in hereditary syphilitics. One also knows how liable they are to the occurrence of morphological anomalies.

In distinction to the organic lesional anxieties, there are the anxieties which I call *psychogenetic*, that is to say those in whom there is no evidence of any organic lesion and in whom, from the fact of the circumstances of life, there are sufficient causes to determine anxiety ; they are the people who have legitimate fears, the difficulties of life.

But the anxiety states also show transitional forms, from the legitimate anxiety to the anxiety which develops the more easily from possible organic anomalies. In psychogenetic anxiety one does not find concomitant pathological manifestations to explain its occurrence.

But, you may say, it is difficult to know whether there may not be dynamic disturbances accountable for the anxiety. This is the reason why I have kept to the last the third variety of anxiety, the one I call *physiogenetic*.

How is one to distinguish these from the psychogenetic anxieties ? In the first place by the general study of the case. It is evident that, when one finds, concomitantly with the anxiety syndrome, distinct sympathetic disturbances, a noticeable instability of the oculo-motor and solar reflexes, vaso-motor disturbances, when there is evidence of sympathetic lability, the chances are in favour of a physiopathic element. In the same way endocrine disturbances, such as hyperthyroidism, make one think of a physiogenetic element.

But all this is fairly hazy ; the personal coefficient often plays an important part. One must therefore replace the impressions of even the most skilled observer, which may be wrong, by objective tests.

It is in this connection that the estimation of hydrogen-ion concentration, by the method of determining the urinary pH, is useful. Let me recall to you how, by Guillaumin's method, one can, by adding a certain quantity of the reagent to a given quantity of urine, estimate the hydrogen-ion concentration. We saw, in the previous lecture, that this hydrogen-ion concentration, when it is increased, is evidenced by a coloration in the urine that varies from yellow to red—as in diabetic acidosis. When the acidosis is diminished, that is to say when the pH is increased, when it passes 6 and reaches 7, there appears, on the contrary, a green coloration, which may be as marked as emerald green. When a pH of 7 is got one can say with certainty that a physiopathic element is present, characterized by a diminution in hydrogen-ion concentration, corresponding to an alkalosis, and which justifies the presence of the anxiety. On this basis, with Cornelius, I believed I had the right to say that there was such a thing as an anxiety, depending on an alkalosis and which one could call an *alkaline anxiety neurosis.*

Thus you appreciate the fact that anxiety, which tends to affect the potentially nervous person who is not tired out, the syndrome which is to the disturbed in mind what asthenia is to the tired out, this kind of " misfire of instinct," has not got only one cause In its mechanism there may or may not enter an endocrine element, but there is always present a sympathetic factor, which sometimes may cause the condition, sometimes only participate in its expression.

I am going to show you now a patient who belongs to this type.

1st Patient.—Mme. Gar——. She is a very simple case, that shows very perfectly the procedure of my concentric method. She is twenty-seven years of age ; sometimes she is somewhat disturbed and nervous. She says that she " is always afraid of falling," that she, " at times has the feeling that she walks on springs." When a car passes her closely at a good pace, she has " the feeling that in passing her very quickly the car will drag her after it."

She has thus a mental syndrome characterized essentially by uneasiness which goes as far as anxiety ; she has, she says, " her heart gripped." From the neurological standpoint, in its sympathetic aspect, we find this well recognized syndrome, that consists of considerable exaggeration of the oculo-cardiac reflex with, on the contrary, absence of the solar reflex. The oculo-cardiac reflex shows a falling away of the pulse from 72 to 36 per minute.

The study of the endocrine zone shows a very definite degree of hyperthyroidism characterized by a goitre, redness of the anterior aspect of the neck, and an enormously increased basal metabolism. On the 6th January last it showed 56,43 large calories instead of 36,5, that is, an increase of over 54 per cent., which certainly indicates a remarkable degree of hyperthyroidism.

Why has Mme. Gar—— hyperthyroidism ? It is possible that here we are dealing with one of these endocrine disturbances so frequent in hereditary syphilitics, for in going well into the history one finds a " morbific kernel " of this order.   M. Hutinel, with his usual masterly skill, has written a remarkable book on the hereditary syphilitic soils.

You see how my concentric method allows one to classify the facts : uneasiness, sensations characterized by a certain number of phobias, emotive function bound up with a sympathetic syndrome of vagal hyper-excitability, without exaggeration of the solar reflex, and signs of hyperthyroidism, in a case of hereditary syphilis.

And this observation leads me to the question, which we must discuss in the next lecture, the question of visceral changes and acquired or hereditary diseases in the psychoneurotic, that is to say the study of the innermost zone, which I call the *morbific kernel*.

VIII

THE ORGANIC DEFECTS AND THE ACQUIRED OR HEREDITARY DISEASES OF THE PSYCHONEUROTIC

THE organic defects and the acquired or inherited diseases of the psychoneurotic constitute in this class of patient what I have termed the *morbific kernel*.

This is a very big question, and I shall only be able to outline it to-day.

Naturally it is necessary to investigate all the possibilities of organic defects before starting on the review of possibilities of either acquired or hereditary disease, and it is only thereafter that one endeavours to arrange the various manifestations noted in their order.

Let me enumerate the various organic defects that must be looked for.

One should pass in review all the possible disturbances of the *respiratory system*, not omitting the nose. Nasal deformities—impairment of freedom of the nasal airways —often play a part in the occurrence of psychoneurotic manifestations. The lung and pleura are important, especially in tuberculous subjects.

In examining the *circulatory system*, one must regard as important not only cardiac disturbances, but also arterial defects, and recognize the part played by early arteriosclerosis, defects of the veins, capillary changes, as well as alterations in the blood itself.

More important still, from the point of view that interests us, are the *digestive disturbances*, not only of the œsophagus, but especially of the stomach, which was the reason why I once said to my former interne Dauptain, when he was beginning his thesis, that one saw almost the same patients in consultation in my service as one found consulting M. Enriquez or attending the gastero-enterology department or M. Gosset's service. It is a fact that a considerable number of patients consult the neurologists for an unrecognized air-swallowing, which has produced a gaseous distension of the stomach and colon. If gaseous distension of the stomach comes to the neurologist chiefly in the form of anxiety, distension of the colon, by the cenesthetic disturbances it causes in the abdomen, is often the cause of true insanities interpreted as hypochrondria, such as one sees in the *reasoning maniacs*.

Here are two cases of this type. Owing to the great clearness of the cause of their troubles, I believe I am justified in demonstrating them to you, although they have both passed the psychoneurotic stage.

1st *Case.*—Mlle. Sophie is a medical student. She has digestive troubles. She says she always has three kinds of spasms, the knots of which, however, are to-day less localized than formerly ; they tie and untie themselves. On my advice she took methylene blue, and felt good effects from it, but only for a very short time, and relapsed back into the "atonic facies." Mlle. Sophie sketches what she feels ; she says " it must be the greater curvature that assumes a small hook-shaped deformity," on account of which the stomach becomes spasmodic, sometimes it has "jolts." In addition to this she says she shows " bulbar phenomena." Now, while the patient feels these sensations at the level of her stomach, the skiagram shows an abnormal condition of the intestine. Indeed she shows a marked degree of *gaseous distension* of the *colon*, chiefly affecting the *splenic flexure*.

The patient also says she has taken atropine sulphate, and that she has suffered from "atonic spasms." Her general state, however, is better ; she has been able to resume her studies. But she says that the cerebral sympathetic takes the "same aspect as the cervical sympathetic," which latter is "held." She says her

" cerebral irrigation " does not work, she " simply can't work," and she eats a great deal. She is less depressed

We advise her to take ergotamine tartrate, of a strength of 1 milgm. in 200 cc. water. She will take one to two teaspoonfuls of this a day.

2nd Case.—This patient, Mme. Maieutique, sixty years of age, has a great faculty of convincing herself of certain things. She says she sees them, and invents nothing

She first consulted my friend Baumgartner, and asked him to operate on her on account of her feeling " a heaviness in the belly which extended in all directions up to her stomach " ; also " she felt she could wait no longer." M. Baumgartner saw her and found absolutely nothing abnormal in her case and told her she was in perfect health. He prescribed a weekly enema with a spoonful of magnesium sulphate. The patient, however, complained that she got worse, but without constipation, fever or skin spots.

But to-day Mme. Maieutique tells us she has noticed something else, a sort of white cyst, like a fine white pearl, and coming from this pearl are seven verdigriscoloured branches ; the longest one reaches the second part of the small intestine, another the rectum. She says she has had a small cancer of the rectum. The other branches were shorter ; in short, the whole thing was like a plant. The seven branches originated in this white cyst, which contained pus, and when this pus escaped it showed as a discharge.

The patient claims she saw all this clearly and the phenomena disappeared under the influence of magnesium sulphate. She adds that she did not see this as one sees a picture, but that it certainly existed and that she saw it in actuality.—This is the phenomenon which M. Sollier has described under the name of autoscopy. The patient says she saw these things with the eyes of the spirit.

Under the influence of magnesium sulphate the branches folded up. But the cyst burst and the pus escaped. She was given belladonna and under its influence the thing shrivelled up, and finally disappeared. It is like a cinema film of plant growth run backwards.

But Mme. Maieutique says that subsequently other phenomena occurred in the neighbourhood of her heart. She saw at the base of the heart a sort of cowl filled with a greenish-brown mass, with hair in the middle of it. It contained also greenish pus. Before she saw this, she says, she felt pain all round her heart, like endocarditis ; she had difficulty in breathing, and it was hard to bend down.

This patient shows, in short, *gaseous distension of the colon*. She eats very little at a time.

The pus then disappeared but the hair remained, and the patient says she saw all this very clearly. She says she is much better, thanks to treatment with iodine and morphine. But every time that a phenomenon disappears there remains a small residuum upon which there develops another poisoning. The patient says she has interrupted her work—she is a good nurse. She claims to be over sixty, though she does not look over fifty. She still complains of slight flushes of warmth, and it is some time since the menstrual function ceased.

As regards the sympathetic system, one notes an exaggeration of the oculo-cardiac reflex.

Consequently the outstanding feature, in this patient, is her very colourful descriptions, which have been discussed, as I told you a moment ago, by Sollier under the name of autoscopic phenomena. Such cases see what happens inside them. Such manifestations have a relationship to their mental reactions and such cases come under the category of the delirious psychopaths, whose limits are establishable between the psychoneurotics and the psychopaths. It is a delirium which corresponds to what used to be described as *internal zoopathy*, but instead of feeling animals in her belly, Mme. Maieutique has the feeling that plants are there. Thus I might call this a delirium of *internal phytopathy*.

These patients develop such states by a process analo-

M

gous to that which one finds in the majority of the psycho-neurotic   Actually this delirium results from a misin-terpretation of cenesthetic sensations.   It is because she has felt curious sensations that this patient has imagined what she has said.   On examining her digestive tube, one notes the presence of *gaseous distension of the colon*, that is to say, the abundant presence of gas in her large intestine, and this condition is of great importance in effecting cenesthetic changes.

This case is very comparable to that of the student who draws the different modifications of her stomach as an omega or an S, according to the drugs she is taking.   The autoscopy of these two women is a product of marked distension of the colon by gas : it is thus by the inter-mediacy of cenesthesia that these patients arrive at the formula of their delirium.   Such distension of the colon attains this importance because of the existence of a mental predisposition, as well as because there is present a hyperæsthesia of cenesthesia ; the student has a vago-sympathetic system of extreme excitability.   One can also, in these cases, establish a diagnosis in depth, and show that, in a way, this delirium is but the *symbolization by the intelligence of cenesthetic sensations arising from visceral disturbances.*

The *gastric, colic, hepatic*, and *renal ptoses* also have a part in the production of the condition, by the dragging which they cause on the solar plexus.

Next we must consider : *disturbances of the pancreas, liver* and *spleen*, since these organs are abdominal, although to be more exact the changes occurring through them should more properly be looked for in the blood.

Disturbances of the Urinary System are also important. Renal cirrhosis, we have already seen as a frequent causative factor in the psychoneuroses of the menopause.

Next, *genital disturbances*, testicular but especially ovarian.

In the *nervous system* the coincidence of changes or definite affections is not very uncommon, and it often indicates a syphilitic heredity. As an example of this I have in private a patient who is not only an absolutely typical case of phobia obsession, but who is also a tabetic from hereditary syphilis, her father dying from cerebral softening due to arteritis, beyond all doubt of luetic origin.

The *osseous system* also shows a series of disturbances which may play a very important part in the production of psychoneurotic manifestations, as may also the *muscular system* and the *integument*.

After this enumeration I am going to show you a case in illustration. She is a patient who will serve as a summary of my previous lecture.

3rd Case.—Mlle. Jeanne. This patient was admitted to the service on account of an anxiety state. She had formerly had an exophthalmic goitre, with such an increase in size of the gland that in 1912 M. Sébileau performed a subcapsular thyroidectomy. At the moment her basal rate is normal and she has a very good scar ; it is a good surgical result. However, she is not completely cured. She has had certain manifestations associated with anxiety and depression which have forced her to give up her work at the Préfecture de la Seine.

She has come under my care, but she has had a series of difficulties, first with one thing then with another ; she believed we wished to do her harm. Formerly, when she was in a convent, she had a belief that pepper was being put in her food to excite her ; she was even the cause of the police being called into the matter, so that the sisters sent her away.

But let us go through Jeanne's history by the concentric method :

First, in the *psychic zone*, there is found a symbolism characterized by æsthetic manifestations which are the very expression of her preoccupations.

She had made symbolic dolls. And each one bears a motto, in which she tells her troubles :

The first doll is Mlle. Chantereine, who bears this title :

"After the great adversities, which have come upon me since 1905, I only desire deliverance, eternal peace, absolute rest." (1924.)

The second doll bears this inscription : " I am crowned with a crown of thorns, whose harsh points have bruised my fragile organs, that will never heal."

Finally, a third doll is Mlle. Roselys, inscribed : "A flower, she, of her own heart, will be both the sympathy and the beauty."

So this patient expresses her unconscious self by æsthetic manifestations ; other cases express theirs in tapestries, which I shall show you and which I owe to my excellent collaborator and friend M. Vichon. Here is an interesting one, which is truly an exteriorization of Freudian conceptions. It was made by a woman suffering from an anxiety at the menopause, who, throughout the course of her life had never sacrificed to Aphrodite; she has depicted a little man in black with a little woman in white who are setting off in each other's company along a road.

Another tapestry contains the story of the asylum where the patient has been under treatment ; she has shown the nurses, the house, etc.

Another one is interesting from the point of view of its colours, in their æsthetic arrangement.

In the same order of ideas is this embroidered canvas, showing all kinds of designs and inscriptions, which is the work of a woman suffering from dementia præcox.

In our patient Jeanne, the psychic zone is characterized not only by æsthetic work but also by evidences of affective transferences. She has an attack of weeping because she says, " they want to take away from her a cat she has picked up and which she says she has already twice saved from death." Thus she has the well-known syndrome of *zoophilia*.

From the psychological standpoint she suffers from intermittent depression with anxiety leading to reactions associated with production of ideas of persecution. Here we are able to see, in a case of chronic anxiety with intermittent periods of depression, the passage of the anxiety syndrome to manifestations of delirium, and her ideas of persecution have produced such social reactions that her life outside an institution has become impossible, and even when she is hospitalized she does anything but make things easy for anyone.

Neurologically, there are no physical signs of organic lesion affection of the nervous system, but there is clearly present a vagosympathetic unbalance, which is always characterized by the same syndrome : considerable exaggeration of the oculo-cardiac reflex with a normal solar reflex.

In the *endocrine* field, Jeanne has chiefly disturbance of ovarian function ; apart from this, with regard to her thyroid, since her operation (in 1912) her basal metabolism is normal.

Viscerally, she has marked disturbance consisting of various ptoses ; the stomach is ptosed and is often the site of spasm ; besides which there is present a syndrome, of frequent occurrence in the depressed, *muco-membranous enterocolitis*.

Finally, if we come to the study of the *morbific kernel*, we find changes relative to an old attack of pulmonary tuberculosis of the right apex.

Thus we are shown to be dealing with a patient suffering from *anxiety and depression with affective repression exteriorized in æsthetic work and in zoophilia, related to a vago-sympathetic imbalance and associated with an endocrine dysfunction, with gastric ptoses and spasm, muco-membranous enterocolitis and signs of old tuberculous lesions of the right apex.*

This case demonstrates the advantage of the concentric method in the diagnosis of the psychoneurotic. And now I am going to select one example from amongst many, to prove the advantage of this method, which allows one to show the facts while leaving the observer entirely free with regard to the discussion of the ætiological order of the manifestations noted.

I come now to an extremely difficult question, that of the interpretation of manifestations of sensitivity, which cannot be controlled objectively, that one sees in the psychoneurotic.

The number of psychoneurotics, who complain of a series of strange disturbances, of variable sensations, which they have difficulty in describing and which correspond very closely to disturbances of cenesthesia, is very large. And the question, which then arises, is to know whether these manifestations are actually felt by the patient or whether they are only the result of delirious ideas showing a mistake in judgment, or whether, indeed, they are related to some organic change that one has not been able to lay bare.

Here are the three possibilities one can consider : is it a question of a true cenestopathy resulting from disturbances of cenesthesia ? or is it a question of *hypochondriac* ideas in the absence of physical signs of organic affection, that is to say the expression of an error of judgment ? or, on the other hand, is it simply the expression of an *organic change?*

At present I have in my service, in the Brouardel ward, three women who, roughly, may be considered to be cenestopaths, that is to say that all three complain of a series of visceral manifestations of the sensitive sort from the head to the feet. Now in each of these three cases there is present changes in the vertebral column ; *the skiagram in all three shows visible change in the spine.*

Let us see whether we can establish a relationship between, on the one hand, the sensitivity manifestations found, and on the other hand the vertebral changes seen.

4th Case.—Mme. Per——. This is the simplest case of the three. She is a woman of fifty-two. *Hereditary antecedents :* Father died at seventy-five ; mother at sixty-seven of a hemiplegia. Husband died at sixty-five at the St. Anne Hospital.

Personal antecedents : When she was twelve years old

she had a fall while jumping a ditch, falling backwards on to her heels; since then she has always had pain in the leg and sacral region. She has had a year in bed with bronchitic trouble; she still suffers with it. She began to menstruate at the age of thirteen. Function has always been regular. In 1918 she had a child, but there is no history of consequent lumbar pain. She had the menopause four years ago. For about the past year the lumbar pains, which never had been entirely absent, have become worse. In point of fact this patient is depressed, with a somewhat increased affectivity, a hypersensibility to noise, insomnia and nightmares. In her dreams, which have been studied by my collaborator, M. Koressios, she says she is often over water, and, as abnormal sensations, she says she has "a feeling like claws on her head, and this feeling extends down her spine; these are not sharp pains, but are like roots gripping in . . . and they also occur in the palate and neck." She feels cracking in her neck, the lumbar and sacral pains have the particular character that they are made worse by walking. "Her heart is often somewhat painful; she feels that her side becomes enormous." She also suffers from "a very great shiveriness."

The objective examination of the nervous system shows normal tendon and pupillary reflexes; sensibility to pain is intact; the vaso-motor streak is perhaps somewhat asymmetrical, less in duration on the right side than on the left. The vertebral column shows slight kyphosis and the most noticeable feature is considerable lumbo-sacral compression. The sacrum is rotated backwards, and the sacro-iliac articulation is the site of lesions that can be very clearly made out in the skiagrams—disappearance of the wing of the sacrum, sacral compression and especially rotation backwards of this bone.

In the cenestopathy one does not find any marked predominance of disturbances at the sacral level. On the contrary the patient shows the condition to be just as well marked at the head level, so one is unable to establish a cause and effect relationship between the two. It is possible that the physical changes may have encouraged the localization of the cenestopathic manifestations to the lower part of the vertebral column, but then they are also found at other levels where there is no indication of any lesion.

5th Case.—This is Mlle. Hen——. I have already shown you this patient in a previous lecture, because she also represents a type on which light is thrown by the concentric method of diagnosis of the psychoneurotic. If we ask this patient to describe her sensations, she will tell us that she feels " a feeling of being enormous, that her body is far from her." She has the impression of an " enormous void " in her body. She says she has pain in her backbone. She feels " as if they were blows with the fist." She suffers " with her whole nervous system " as if she had " a motor car stopped, with the engine running normally." She has drawn a diagram to show how her whole body is compressed by her sympathetic. And this starts chiefly at the lower end of her digestive tube. In addition she says " she hears her thoughts resonate everywhere, to the right and the left."

She has the feeling that she is " outside her body." Her diagram illustrates her troubles of vision ; she " has a black point which turns continually." When she walks she has " the feeling that her body is much bigger than it actually is." This diagram is a *symbolization* of her judgment of the manifestations which she feels.

Now, let us look at the skiagrams. First take the skull : nothing abnormal there unless it be calcification of the Pacchionian bodies. The skiagram of the vertebral column shows a *dorso-lumbar scoliosis*.

Do these slight disabilities of the vertebral column play a part of any sort in the causation of the general cenesto-pathic manifestations which this patient describes ? Certainly not. There is no cause and effect relationship between the two. For when she speaks she immediately confuses the psychic manifestations with those of somatic expression ; one really gets the impression that both of these are only the symbolizations of her judgment on what is occurring in her, so that we are really dealing here with an *imaginative symbolism*, with interpretations of these organic sensations as psychic phenomena taking place within her ; and it would be straining the facts to want to find, in the coincidental occurrence of a slight scoliosis, a satisfactory cause of the localization or even the causality of the cenestopathic manifestations.

6th Case.—Mme. Am——. This is a woman of fifty-seven years who has a positive family history : a father somewhat alcoholic, a mother who died at sixty-nine, who was nervous and who treasured a marked dislike for the patient ; one deceased brother suffered from diabetes.

Personal history : At the age of seventeen months, she fell into the fire, after which she must have begun to speak. At seven she had paratyphoid fever. She menstruated at twelve. She has had three children. Before she was forty-five she was nervous, but after that age and especially since her menopause, which occurred at forty-eight, she has shown painful phenomena of the head and spine. In 1912 she consulted M. Gilbert Ballet for these pains in the head and constant giddiness. In 1915, while suffering from periods of anxiety, she was treated by M. G. Ballet by laudanum. In 1916 she saw M. Dupré for an old state of depression, with remissions, cenestopathy, aches, and a hypochondriac state.

In 1920, I examined her ; her blood pressure with the Pachon machine showed hypertension ; I gave her benzyl benzoate. Her blood-pressure [1] fell from 25 to 19.10 ; the pulse is between 92 and 100. At that time she suffered from a *spasmodic coryza*. In 1926 she came back to see me ; she was very depressed. At the present time, she still is. She stays nearly the whole time in bed, in order to avoid disagreeable sensations, which she says she feels

[1] See footnote on p. 44.

more when she is up. Her affectivity is exaggerated ;
she easily becomes irritable, by crises, which appear to be
related to a hypersensibility caused by certain preoccupations, which she has for her illness. " I would like
to die, there isn't a minute when I don't suffer . . ."
from which she draws the conclusion : " I must be made
of granite to be able to stand up to such suffering ! " This
reaction of pride is common in hypochondriacs.

At first, the thing that helped her most was massage.
But she says that she is suffering again, and even to-day
she says she has pains " everywhere, in the backbone and
in the head," she says she feels as if " something torments
and irritates her. . . ."

She dreams a lot, and her dreams have been fully studied
by Koressios. She feels herself lifted up into space, sus-
pended in the void, that she makes movements with her
arms and flies. . . . It is certainly true that she has an
exaggerated sensibility. The particular sensations that
annoy and irritate her more exasperate her than they
give her pain. She says they are " intolerable." Light
and noise upset her ; " I should like to be in the dark,"
she says. Since her menopause she has sensations of
" beating, swinging, and oscillations in her brain." She
claims she has a cerebral congestion with a reflection at
the level of her vertebral column, a condition that worries
and depresses her. She feels in her spine " something like
small gravel sticking, especially in the lower part of the
vertebral column " ; this gravel collects and even the
touch of her underclothing becomes a great annoyance
in her bad periods." She feels the cold badly, and she
says that at the start she felt her vertebral column " very
cold like ice."

Palpation brings on an attack of annoyance, and she
becomes unstable emotionally. She says that she sometimes feels in her left leg " that the flesh is coming off
the bone," and she has the feeling also that her leg is
" made of glass " . . . she always has a feeling of being
cold.

The treatment she is receiving sometimes causes her abnormal sensations. Iodema, which M. Thiroloix found to give excellent results in chronic rheumatism, gave her a bitter taste, and did not have a beneficial effect on this patient.

I have tried diathermy on the painful parts, but it was no more productive of a beneficial effect.

She also says she feels her heart is getting bigger, and she shows dyspnœa. She has had digestive troubles. Her general condition, however, is normal : pulse is 80, lungs are normal.

The vertebra column shows changes between the eleventh and twelfth dorsal vertebræ, which would seem to indicate ossification of the intervertebral cartilaginous disc. The skiagram also shows the presence of " parrot beaks " in the lower and upper parts of the vertebræ.

Thus, from the X-ray appearances, one may describe the state of this patient as follows :

An intervertebral lesion between D 11 and D 12 ; antero-posterior and lateral views normal. The superior surface of the body of the 12th dorsal vertebra is not the same as the inferior aspect of the body of the 11th. They enclose between them a fusiform space, which is occupied by the intervertebral meniscus, whose centre would appear to be ossified. This rare condition has been described by Calvé. A fresh and more close examination, however, did not show this to be present.

The study of the nervous system shows an asymmetry of cutaneous sensibility when objectively controlled. Pain sensibility is increased in that part of the body beneath a line running obliquely outwards and downwards from the 10th dorsal vertebra.

We find the objectively controlled disturbances correspond to the vertebral rheumatoid condition, which we have already noted. The temperature sense is not disturbed to heat, but in contrast we find a general hyperesthesia to cold ; the cold tube is felt as ice.

You notice that this case is much more complex than

the others. We note in this patient three kinds of disturbance.

1. A definite *chronic rheumatism*, with special sensations and particularly disturbance of objectively controlled sensibility corresponding to the vertebral lesions. Consequently there is present a *vertebro-neurological association*.

2. In this patient there are *hypochondriac preoccupations associated with a state of periodic depression ;* she localizes this not only in her head but also in her lower extremities or at the level of the vertebral column. Consequently these disturbances, of which she complains, are more extensive than the objective vertebral manifestations noted.

Is this a reason for crediting all the manifestations of which she complains to the account of disturbances of judgment of a hypochondriac nature ? I do not believe so. I believe that we have here, in addition to the hypochondriac preoccupations, a form of the syndrome which Dupré has described under the name of cenestopathy. The multiplicity of their descriptions, apart from their character, which remains more or less the same, whoever the patient may be, clearly shows that it is not merely a question of the imaginative structure erected by a judgment that is trying to interpret only an uneasiness. Something is present which appears to originate in disturbance of cenesthesia. And it is conceivable that granted the lesions we have noted, and knowing, on the other hand, that *compression of the rami communicantes* is capable of causing cenesthetic disturbances, it is possible to establish a cause and effect relationship between the chronic rheumatism and some degree of the cenesthesia.

I believe, then, that this case enables us to explain, naturally not completely but at least partially, the predominant localization of some of the preoccupations of this patient.

Thus you see how much the question of relationship between the sympathetic disturbances and the psychic expressions and also the relationship between the sympathetic disturbances and the objective facts relating to the different viscera or systems, demand a detailed neurological examination in each particular case.

If, now, I complete the analysis of this *morbific kernel*, I must review all the diseases that may play a part in causality of such accidents. First come the infectious diseases, which most commonly of all play a part in these cases, beginning with the diseases of childhood. One must regard, as one of the most important, *scarlet fever*, which is very liable to affect the endocrine glands, and consequently frequently causes psychoneuroses. Then come diphtheria, typhoid fever, and paludism, whose part in the origination of psychoneuroses has been shown during the war, in the Eastern theatres, by my friend Vinchon. Then tuberculosis, epidemic encephalitis, syphilis, alcoholism, high blood uric acid and high oxalæmia, which easily lead to vago-sympathetic changes. Then come those processes which lead to acidosis, alkalosis, and avitaminosis, and amongst tumours, particularly fibromata.

And now I come to the morbific kernel originating in hereditary diseases. At the head of this list I would place syphilis, either in the first, second or third generation ; and then hereditary alcoholism.

Having thus analysed the five zones, one must study the ætiological order. This depends on multiple factors. Once the symptoms are known it becomes a question of establishing their *relationships*—of *causality, interdependence,* or whether they are only simple *coincidences.* But even when one only finds the simple relationship of coincidence, it has to be borne in mind, if one cannot show evidence of a *physiological relationship*, that one ought always to consider the possibility of *psychological relationships.*

A person who has gross organic defects, who is a cripple, or very ugly, or who, from a restricted range of movement of the arms, has a loss of his social capacity, may secondarily, from the fact of the bitterness resulting from his incapacity, show psychoneurotic manifestations, which, in such a case, are not explicable physiologically, but can be accounted for psychologically, and it is only having gone through the different zones, psychic, neurological, endocrine, visceral and morbific, that one can establish a treatment, which, by the same token, must be social, humoral, neurological, sympathetic, endocrine, visceral, and lastly ætiological.

And to conclude, I shall take a very particular example, which I have called the *hypotensive endocrino-neurosis*. I shall show you how, in this case, one can apply the big general principles, which I have tried to bring before you to-day. This will be the subject of my next lecture.

IX

SYMPTOMS, DIAGNOSIS, AND TREATMENT OF HYPOTENSIVE ENDOCRINONEUROSIS

I AM giving this lecture on a somewhat particular type of endocrinoneurosis to show afresh the usefulness of the *concentric method* for the classification of symptoms, found by clinical observation, without being obliged to arrange them beforehand in their ætiological order.

This is a clinical type, which generally puzzles many observers, who are more or less wittingly attached by the anatomical habit of thought to the old division of the neuropaths, because in this type there is such a diffusion into the different sympathetic fields that it becomes extremely difficult to show the presence of a lesion localized to one of the glands of internal secretion.

Before making the synthesis of the symptomatology of the hypotensive endocrinoneurosis, I believe it will be advisable to read you a part of the case history of a patient I am attending in private, given by herself, who belongs to this type which we have already seen in Mlle. Sylvie C——, who in the clinical analysis of her surface manifestations showed elements of hysteria, neurasthenia, psychasthenia, and emotive psychoneurosis.

Here, very briefly, is the history of this patient :

" She is an unmarried woman of twenty-seven, of gouty diathesis, who had, at the age of seven, scarlet fever ; keep that in mind. From the age of five to fourteen she had, almost regularly, every month, attacks of migraine which ended in vomiting. She began menstruating at fourteen and a half, and from this time on one may say that she has always been tired. Also about the same time she showed a scoliosis, of slight degree, but which is still apparent.

" Her growth has been irregular ; for the first few years she was quite small, then she suddenly began to grow, about the time of puberty.

" The pathological manifestations began, one might say, with digestive troubles, which is a frequent occurrence in such patients. At first they were mostly cramps, and spasms. A series of gastric analyses was done for hyperchlorhydria. She was treated in Bern by Prof. Dubois, in his sanatorium, with abundant diet and massage of the stomach, and put on a few kilos.

" Then, having made some improvement for two or three months, after some further time the same treatment produced the opposite effect, and Sylvie felt worse. She lost weight progressively ; she became sensitive to cold and depressed. The digestive troubles changed their character. Intestinal fermentation appeared. She became extremely sensitive to changes of temperature ; on the least provocation she caught sore throat. She also complains of acne eruptions, and it appears that these are related to the unhealthy state of her alimentary tract and the irregularity of her menstrual function, which is small in amount, often late, and frequently ' missing months '."

Such is the history in a few words up to the last few months and she has completed these observations by several supplementary details which she has given me.

She has consulted many physicians, and as a rule this is what happens ; a new physician, new treatment, and during the first few weeks that follow she improves ; then in a short time she becomes less well and in a way she has a relapse that sends her back to where she was before.

In addition, Sylvie gives such heed to her diet that if one article of food causes some small discomfort, she suppresses it and so comes to diminish her total intake.

This is a point to which Jean Charles Roux has called attention—the frequency of undernourishment in neuropaths, who, fearing to cause upset by certain articles of diet, end by almost cutting out all their diet. Of course at one time someone had put her on a purely vegetarian diet. She then noted that when she went back to proteins, she had a series of continued manifestations, violent cephalalgy, vomiting, and skin eruptions, as if the influence of the ingestion of new albumins had produced a phenomenon somewhat resembling anaphylaxis.

Then the digestive disturbances became continually dominant, and by dint of palpation, Sylvie came to have a somewhat tender right iliac fossa, and the question arose as to whether these manifestations were not related to a chronic appendicitis. The appendix was removed. The remarkable fact was that, as is the rule in these patients, although she appeared extremely delicate and on the least medication showed extraordinary reactions, Sylvie stood the shock of operation perfectly well. The anæsthesia, the operation and the postoperative period were uneventful and the whole affair was over in fifteen days.

But during the two or three weeks which followed, the general condition, which had appeared to have undergone improvement, became less favourable and the other disturbances soon reappeared.

At the present time this patient still complains of spasms at the level of the stomach, of pain after food, intestinal fermentation, constipation, and this fatigue which had always accompanied the condition.

But one must not think that this patient, who has been seen by some thirty doctors, has not been well examined, and that a finger has not been placed on the most important point in the determinism of her troubles. Thus an excellent confrère has made the diagnosis of hysteroneurasthenia of endocrine origin, with adrenal insufficiency, thyro-ovarian insufficiency, intestinal ptosis, dyspepsia, intestinal fermentation, dry pleurisy, pleuro-pulmonary affections, cardiac murmur—which of course corresponds to our concentric method of diagnosis of psychoneurotics.

Sylvie's temperature is normal. A very interesting

N

point is that she says that her throat is very delicate ; she has noticed that when her throat is inflamed, her digestive tube is better ; and in addition when a sore throat is coming on she has a better appetite than usual.

It is very interesting thus to see the manifestations of vagotonia, which these are, caught in full light by the patient herself. It is obvious that she is ignorant of the physiology of these details, and of vagus function. Her observations have all the greater value for that reason. It is an example of the transference of metastases so common in vagotonics, which has given rise to the theory of metastases which Broussais stresses.

When a sore throat is coming on she says she is hungrier than ordinarily ; this is due to hyperexcitability of the vagus which will go on to painful and inflammatory manifestations of the naso-pharynx.

To complete this clinical picture, the patient has not only attacks of migraine, but she is also subject to crops of urticaria.

From this observation it becomes clearly evident that there are present sympathetic disturbances, chiefly characterized by a vagus hyperexcitability together with an endocrine disturbance, dominated by adrenal insufficiency and hypogonadism.

This clinical picture is confirmed by examination of the urine, whose specific gravity is 1010, due to deficiency in elimination, dependent on under-nourishment, with a pH of 7, that is a rise in the figure indicating alkalosis. The twenty-four hourly urea is 1.57, indicating a diminished protein intake ; the uric acid was quite large in amount at 0.53 cgr. ; there was a very distinct urinary hypo-acidity with a high blood uric acid.

The basal metabolism was of interest in view of the endocrine complexity. It is characterized by a diminution. The patient is very thin but seems at times to show signs of hyperthyroidism. Actually she has a slight hypofunction with a basal metabolism of 36.6 calories, or in other words 3.9 per cent. below normal.

Elicitation of the sympathic reflexes shows very clearly exaggeration of the solar reflex, which is very strongly positive ; there is a diminution of the amplitude of the oscillations on applying epigastric compression. With regard to the oculo-cardiac reflex, a priori one would have expected it to be exaggerated, considering that there is a normally slow pulse—between 60 and 64 ; now, this reflex, elicited by M. Largeau, only gave a slowing of from 64 to 56, or 8 beats a minute. It would thus appear to be normal, but I believe that the ocular compression was not strongly enough applied, and in addition a normal or only slightly positive response does not allow one to form the opinion that the vagus is not somewhat hyperexcitable.

This example, briefly cited, on information got this morning from the patient, will enable us to place the *clinical type*, which I want to bring before you systematically, by reviewing seriatim the five zones, in order to make the psychoneurotic diagnosis according to the concentric method, which I have taught you to apply.

First, then, the *general aspect*. As a rule the patients are women. Up till now I have not met this clinical type in men. Also they are chiefly young women or young unmarried women, who are tall and thin, and in whom the neck is often very long, and using this artistic criterion one can in a fashion make a retrospective diagnosis of hypotensive endocrinoneurosis. In Florence you can see in the Santa Maria Novella, on the right-hand wall behind the High Altar, a fresco by Guirlandajo, which is a portrait of Simonetta Tornabuoni, which shows some of the features I have just mentioned, and who died of tuberculosis. You recall the descriptive appearance of our patient, who is also to some extent tuberculous. Simonetta Tornabuoni had this same long, cylindrical neck, which had made such an impression on Botticelli that most of his Madonnas are of this type ; the Primavera incidentally also died of tuberculosis.

These patients show also a great fatigability. They

show such hyperæsthesia that those about them tend to
think their sensations are purely imaginary. Coexistent
with this are a hypercenesthesia and a defective differentiation between the manifestations of the superficial self
of consciousness and the unconscious self, as well as a
certain degree of lack of differentiation between the
sensory-motor manifestations and those of the sympathetic,
as if the subjects were still in the infantile state. This
being the general aspect, let us now study these cases,
and analyse the different zones.

First, the psychic zone.—Let us first clear the psychic
zone of all the reactional contingent manifestations of the
psychic state, which is the expression of deeper manifestations. In this clearing up, we must first eliminate
all the familial interpsychological reactions, which play
a very important part, the parents reacting according to
their characters to the manifestations in the sick person,
and the patient often becoming the centre of all familial
activity, from which arises a multiplication of the symptoms from the attention given to what the patient suffers
by the parents. So it often happens that the most carefully directed treatment is of no effect so long as the patient
is not isolated from her familial surroundings.

Then there are the episodic psychological reactions
which come from changes in the cenesthetic state, reactions of discouragement with periods of euphoria
which are dependent on changes in a nervous state that
is essentially labile. One must emphasize the instability
of the nervous state, and these reactions take their tone
from the contingent situation. This is the reason why
one is able, in these patients, depending on the time and
the personal orientation to find that they belong more or
less to the hysterical picture, the neurasthenic, psychasthenic, or emotive psychoneurotic pictures, as I had
occasion to point out in dealing with the patient I showed
you in the first lecture.

Then, in the third place, this psychic atmosphere, consisting chiefly of a state of emotion, of feelings, of tenden-

cies resulting from the diffuse cenesthetic state, leads very easily, by a classical process, if not to an appearance of insanity, at least to fancied interpretations derived from conditions of environment and civilization. This is why one sees all the transitions up to insanity more or less systematized ; this is how it happens that some patients when seen by psychiatrists are considered as properly called hypochondriacs, and when seen by other people are considered as possessed ; and so we can see all these types with the clinical picture character of the possessed.

Having rid the patient of his more or less insane interpretations, secondary insane reactions and familial interpsychological reactions, one tackles the psychic zone proper, and first studies the *superficial social aspect*.

From this point of view here is a frequent occurrence : the relatives, father, mother, sisters, or brothers, say of the patient—she's lazy, she can't do a thing. This is important, and indicates deep disturbances, related in this particular case to adrenal insufficiency. Laumonier had the merit of showing the *frequency of laziness in adrenal insufficiency.*

In addition these are women who seem to be cold, unemotive, without marked reactions in their emotions ; the relatives say they feel nothing. Now, just the opposite is true. These are the children or young girls who have a considerable hyperaffectivity, that is characterized by an emotive hypoeffectivity, due to the fact that their sympathetic does not have an extremely enhanced tonus.

The adolescent or the child grows at an unequal rate— by bursts of growth. This growth in spurts is operative not only in the general state but also in the particular systems, and at adolescence these young girls may show dysharmony related to some degree of dyspituitarism and which finds expression in a subacromegaly.

From the social aspect these cases show depression, periods of anxiety with pithiatic reactions and sometimes stronger manifestations

And this brings me to the analysis of the *unconscious self*.

The essential characteristic of this unconscious self is, one might say, *hypercenesthesia*. They are patients who have what one might call hypertrophy of their cenesthesia ; the cenesthetic manifestations which at first in the depth of the being are covered by the successive sensory-motor layers, come to the surface of consciousness. From this results a very great facility of observation and the tendency to attach too great importance to variations in affectivity. This very easily becomes a more or less superstitious state, reinforced by the frequency of intuitions. When this happens in people of little developed intelligence, they skip in a way the discursive intelligence, to arrive directly at their impressions and judgment. Such intuitions are characterized by the frequency of *premonitions*. Frequently these patients have presentiments, apparently really derived from the collection in their unconscious self of a series of signs which escape their conscious senses.

Without going as far as the cryptæsthesia of Prof. Ch. Richet, it is undoubtedly true that in these people one notes a series of premonitions that appear to indicate that they guess right a greater number of times than the law of probabilities would appear to indicate as likely. The manifestations of these premonitions lie in the interpretation of their dreams, " *onirocriticism.*" And very often, in these patients, one finally gets in their dreams the proof of the sensibility of their unconscious self.

There results from this that such people are particularly liable to two manifestations, which have for long interested psychiatrists. These are mediumship and mysticism. It is evident that it is from the ranks of these patients that many mediums and mystics are recruited.

Neurological Zone.—Here we must study the sensory-motor aspect before passing to the sympathetic.

There are some very remarkable manifestations in the sensory-motor aspect—from the sensory point of view I refer to olfactory hyperæsthesia. This olfactory hyper-acuity is periodic in its occurrence and degree ; it is exaggerated under the influence of the beginning of pregnancy, for example, and I think it very likely that it is related to a vagus hyperexcitability. I shall not go into details here on the anatomical considerations, that can be given in explanation of this. But M. Nicholas has described at the base of the brain a small nerve, the *cerebral nerve*, which is found in the neighbourhood of the olfactory nerve and appears to have connections with the sympathetic system. It is also certain that as the mam-mals evolve towards the human type, the olfactory system diminishes in size (this system has been fully studied by Broca). It is evident that in creatures lower in the scale than mammals there is a general olfactory system, while as one rises in the scale this system tends to become of less importance. You see in this a fact analogous to what I said at the beginning in connection with these patients, that there is in them a defect of differentiation.

In addition to this everyone is familiar with the close relationship between perfumes and sex. Also these patients are great lovers ; they have hypergonadism and a considerable development of their genital functions. Consequently all this is quite compatible. Apart from this, this hyperæsthesia is not the only thing that occurs. There is also a hyperalgesia much greater in extent than what is found in normal subjects ; one must therefore not consider the hypotensive endocrinoneurotic as soft and cowardly ; they have a lowered threshold of pain sensibility.

From the motor point of view, the essential character-istic of these cases is *muscular hypotonus*, which appears to be more than a nervous modification, an actual physical condition of their muscle fibres. They show a general lack of tone, not only of the striped muscle and indicated by the poor development of their musculature but also laxity of ligaments, so that one can dorsiflex their fingers to an angle of 90 degrees. Also the poor tone of plain muscle explains the frequency of *varicose veins* in these cases.

In addition the tonus of their arteries is poor. On auscultation one hears very little vibratory hum. They readily feel upset if they suddenly change their position because their muscular tone is unable immediately to compensate gravity effects.

From the sensory-motor aspect, then, one must note *hyperæsthesia* and a certain degree of *hypotonia*.

Sympathetic aspect.—This can be summarized in two conditions : a quite remarkable *hypercenesthesia* and a *vagotonia*. Let us examine these two points.

From the vaso-motor point of view these patients are apt to show *acrocyanosis* ; the extremities are cold and cyanotic, and in some of them this leads to a certain degree of shyness. They fear they appear ugly. There is a true *phobia of ugliness*. The nose is often blue ; they are liable to chilblains and scaling of the tip of the nose. In addition these vaso-motor disturbances lead to variations in the volume of limbs, due to changes in position ; if they remain for long on their feet their legs swell. This defect in tone also is responsible for changes in volume of the extremities in relation to the menstrual function. Many of them have a fullness of the belly for a few days before the period ; changes also occur in the size of the hands. While they are still some little way from a period their rings fall off their fingers—like Mélisande's, but during the period the fingers are swollen, and show grooves made by the rings which can be no longer taken off.

These defects in tonus, then, related to vaso-motor disturbances, produce, on the one hand, a tendency to a hypothymic state, and on the other, a tendency to urticaria, which be it noted is a manifestation which is not of the same category as the presence of dermography ; one may, indeed, find cases of hypotensive endocrino-neurosis who show urticarial but not dermographic manifestations.

In connection with the sympathetic reactions, one must also note the relative frequency of migraine.

Unstriped-muscle phenomena are also in evidence ; these are the cases who are unable to go long without food, are constipated with spasmodic conditions that result therefrom, and have as well a general state of ptosis ; and these *ptoses* produce a secondary excitability of the sympathetic chain by dragging on the solar plexus.

As regards pilo-motor function, such cases are usually cold, but rarely show " gooseflesh," which on the contrary one does find in those suffering from hyperorthosympathicotonia.

The secretory function shows one cold in the head after another, and sneezing fits occur with the least change of temperature ; very often this syndrome is present due to *stimulation of the sphenopalatine ganglion.*

From the trophic point of view, one notes some fragility of the skin, also some degree of instability of body weight ; such women easily change weight. This *instability in weight* is partly due to change in body volume ; the changes in density are related to the vaso-motor disturbances of which I have already spoken.

Endocrine Zone.—Here one must inspect both the morphological and humoral aspects.

Morphological aspect.—These patients have large hands and to some extent the appearance of *dissociated acromegaly.* The head shows hypertrichosis ; a light shadow can be seen on the upper lip, such as Flaubert describes in Emma Bovary. Their hair is " electric," it crackles when combed with a tortoiseshell or celluloid comb ; in the dark it gives off sparks, which may have been the foundation of the idea of the halo of the saints. This falls in the category of the phenomena of illumination of the saints studied by the mystics in Ribet's very remarkable book on divine mysticism in which one finds a number of examples of the phenomena of radiance. This certainly is a fact—that there is a relationship between hagiography and the experimental occurrence of these phenomena in certain psychoneurotics.

The neck is more or less cylindrical in form, indicating some degree of thyroid trouble, the smallness of the neck coinciding with a condition of hypothyroidism. However this does not in any way preclude the occurrence of intermittent reactional crises of hyperthyroidism in an organ whose general level is hypofunctional.

When there is hypothyroidism, the torso shows small breasts. This is indeed the rule in subjects who are hyperovarian, which fact is not contradictory to the excellence of lactation, and one may say that these women with small breasts are as a rule good nurses.

While one is noting this special appearance of the torso one often sees at the same time that there is some scoliosis present.

The abdomen as a rule shows ptoses. When these women are seen nude an infra-umbilical sinking in is apparent, or on the other hand the lower part of the abdomen may be somewhat rounded, as in the Eve of Jan and Hubert van Eyck. This is related to some hypotonicity of the muscles of the abdominal wall, which is not well developed.

The lower limbs are generally fairly long, due to a relatively late puberty and because there has been overgrowth of the lower extremities, which is generally the rule in the hypogonad. Also these legs are very often covered with hair.

Humoral aspect.—I have been able to find a series of changes that allows one to classify the various endocrine disturbances. Examination of the blood : hypoglycæmia, hypoadreninæmia, hypocholersterinæmia, and pH over 7, indicating alkalosis.

Analysis of the adrenal functions shows marked insufficiency with *hypoadreninæmia* and *hypocholesterinæmia.* On the other hand there is present in the adult, from the time of organic puberty, hyperovarianism with hypertrichosis ; menorrhagia ; small breasts, active sex life and very good pregnancies. This is an important point to note, that pregnancy is excellent in these patients and lactation is exhausting. This detail should be kept in mind—one should beware of lactation, for it entails a considerable loss of calcium. Now, as these patients have already a low blood calcium, a too prolonged lactation aggravates this and leads to sympathetic excitability, which predisposes them to a lighting up of the tuberculous condition.

There is a dyspituitarism, characterized by disproportionate growth of the extremities, which occurs in slight degree reactively first in one direction then in the other so that it is hard to say whether the gland is overactive or underactive—one can only say that there is " disturbed " function. Another endocrine instability is characterized by hypothyroidism with paroxysmal crises of relative hyperthyroidism, so that sometimes these patients seem to be suffering from Basedow's disease. These are *false Basedows with paroxysmal periods of relative reactional hyperthyroidism on a hypothyroid basis*. This has been definitely noted by my good friend Léopold Lévy with H. de Rothschild in their study of the endocrine glands.

From the point of view of the parathyroids, one finds a low blood calcium. Now, one knows that in tetany, which is connected with low blood calcium, there is a relationship to parathyroid insufficiency, and this seems to me to play a part in the frequent appearance of anxiety in these patients. Then in some cases I would be ready to believe that there may be a too high blood insulin, that these patients have a somewhat overactive pancreas. In spite of a frequent and relative adiposity of the lower extremities, they are thin, eat well, but don't get fat, owing to the fact of an overactive pancreas, which causes destruction of all the carbohydrate elements. The possibility occurs to one of this high blood insulin playing a part in the phenomena of anxiety, for after insulin injections, even with the most protein-free preparations, when the patient has not taken beforehand a sufficient amount of carbohydrate, there is often an attack of anxiety due to a transitory hyperinsulinæmia.

This same description, from this point of view, resembles the facts which my good friend and colleague Gougerot noted a few years ago, when he described a special form of endocrine dysfunction under the name of *hyperinsulinæmia*.

Visceral Zone.—One must examine separately the functional aspect and the anatomo-pathological aspect.

Functional aspect.—This is either the reflection or the concomitant of the cause of some part of the sympathetic manifestations noted. Thus at the head of the list of functional visceral disturbances one must place disturbances of the alimentary tract ; this is why, as my pupil Dauptain very rightly said in his thesis, one sees in my service more or less the same patients as in the services dealing specially with diseases of the digestive system. In these cases there is seen bulimy or anorexia, with reduction of the diet for fear of pain, producing undernourishment. In severer cases one may find mental anorexia with its very serious consequences.

Also there is found extremely frequently *ptosis* of the stomach and colon with the symptoms depending on whether they are total or, which is more frequent, from the point of view of positive sympathetic reactions, when there is prolapse of the transverse colon, when *Lane's syndrome* is found. From the fact that the colic flexures become progressively more acute angled, instead of being right angled, the passage of contents becomes very difficult, produces secondary spasms, and peripheral reactions of the orthosympathetic, characterized by extreme coldness of the hands and feet, so much so that Lane finds the handshake almost diagnostic.

Intermittent and reactional spasms also appear, which are not incompatible with the condition of ptosis, which seem often to be complicated by air swallowing with distension of the stomach, which presses against the heart and causes crises of anxiety, and gaseous distension of the colon, which, by abdominal discomfort and changes in the cenesthesia resulting from this embarrassment of the transverse colon and particularly its splenic flexure, may become a source of excitation of insane interpretations. We saw an example of this in the woman student who suffers from systematized reasoning insanity, related to *gaseous distension of the colon*, and accompanied, as often happens, by secondary constipation due to excitability of the vagus system.

Dropped kidney, especially on the right side, and prolapse of the womb may also be found.

The *Circulatory System*. Cardiac anxiety with palpitations and tachycardia, to account for which investigation should be directed to the digestive system or vagosympathetic. Varicosities are also frequent as are acromegalic evidences.

The *Respiratory System* should be carefully examined. One notes predisposition to tuberculosis.

In the *Urinary System*, one is struck by the fact that these patients drink very little fluid, that is to say that owing to their low pressure, they are never thirsty, drink therefore very little, and, as a consequence, pass a urine which is insufficient to eliminate all their waste products. As a result there is some intoxication present, due to insufficient elimination.

The *Genital System* is interesting in that there is often some degree of hyperovarian function and an active sex life. Such disturbances as are characterized by leucorrhœa are also of frequent occurrence.

The *General State of Nutrition* is also worthy of note, for these patients readily show *anaphylactic* manifestations. I shall not go into detailed descriptions ; the body fluids are liable to flocculence depending on the nature of the food ingested, and depending on the humoral state which is closely connected with physical disposition ; but what is certain, from the nutritional viewpoint, is that these patients have great difficulty in putting on flesh. There is, then, difficulty in putting on weight, fluctuations in weight, and subnormal temperature, 35 degrees to 36 degrees C. Sometimes under the influence of over-fatigue the temperature may touch 37 or over, but it soon falls to 35 or 36.

In the *Muscular* and *Cutaneous Systems*, loss of tone is observed.

The skin is delicate with a tendency to urticaria. In the *Skeletal System*, there is a tendency to scoliosis.

Anatomo-pathological aspect.—Behind the functional disturbances of the digestive system one must be sure that there is not an ulcer, pyloric or duodenal, or that there is not a duodenal diverticulum or a condition of peri-visceritis. It was to Carnot's credit that he drew attention to the frequency of *perivisceritis*, and it is certain that *adhesions* play an important part in the disturbances affecting passage of bowel contents, particularly in the abdominal sympathetic reactions.

Also, a sharp look-out must be kept for the occurrence of *biliary lithiasis*, there is a vicious circle of vagotonia and hepatic colic. Certainly vagotonia, such as occurs premenstrually, facilitates the appearance of these phenomena, and biliary lithiasis by the local vagotonia it produces may play a part in general changes.

From the viewpoint of circulatory changes, one notes the frequency of " cœur en goutte," heart sounds that are heard like falling drops.

In the respiratory system, the frequency of tuberculous lesions should be noted.

In the urinary system, the frequency of lithiasis, particularly *oxalate stone.*

Morbific Kernel.—Let us first consider the acquired diseases. Two of those play a very important part ; *scarlet fever* and *diphtheria.* Léon Bernard and Bigard have drawn attention to this fact of adrenal insufficiency produced by experimental diphtheritic intoxication.

Clinically one may cite the frequency of hypoadrenalism after diphtheria, which causes a post-diphtheria vagotonia.

On the other hand scarlet fever, which seems particularly to affect the endocrine glands, by the post-scarletinal endocrine disturbance it produces, causes scoliosis.

Regarding *Hereditary Diseases*, there is one which plays a considerable part here and to which sufficient attention is not usually given—*Gout*. It seems likely that many of these patients have a gouty diathesis and that such familial defence reactions are established, as are usually chiefly found in the psychological field, but which are found here also and which may be compared with the adages : " Miserly father, prodigal son," " Perfectly balanced father, unbalanced son," etc. In the same way as one sees the evolution of reaction in different branches of the same family, for the establishment of an equilibrium which subsequently is attained, I believe there to be similar changes in the organism. I have very often observed the descendants of gouty people extraordinarily strong and robust, defying the years and living to a great age, in turn giving rise to people of feeble health who die prematurely; and these descendants of the gouty are apt to have a high blood oxalate, that is to say they assimilate oxalic acid with difficulty, and this oxalate retention plays an important part in these cases by causing a certain degree of anxiety through vagus excitation. This is why one must forbid them chocolate.

There is also the *alcoholic* diathesis, the *syphilitic* diathesis which so often affects the endocrine glands ; and the *tuberculous diathesis*.

Having said this with reference to the *static state* of these patients, let us now study their evolution.

Evolution.—Their evolution is in spurts. We have said, in connection with the genital system, that the pregnancies were excellent and the lactation exhausting. The dominant feature seems to be *adrenal insufficiency and hyperovarianism*, as well as a predisposition to pulmonary tuberculosis.

Summarizing, we have to deal with a syndrome characterized by hypercenesthesia with vagotonia related to an adrenal insufficiency and hyperovarianism, with vicarious pituitary and thyroid reactions, occurring in people who are disproportionately overgrown in their long bones, suffer from scoliosis, poor musculature, ptoses, poor heart action, and who are vagotonic, hyperaffective, and relatively unemotive. This condition often arises as the result of scarlet fever in the hereditarily gouty, in families of unstable thyroid tendency.

The diagnosis that may be made in them varies with whichever zone symptoms, which we have studied, dominate the clinical picture. It may be a diagnosis of hysteria, of neurasthenia, of hypochondria, or of Basedow's disease, in which there are various disturbances of the ovarian, adrenal, and pituitary functions ; or it may be a diagnosis of ptosis, or even of organic affections of the digestive system, of cutaneous affections, renal, genital, or nervous affections ; and this brings me to the treatment.

Treatment.—Naturally this must depend on the various indications in the different zones.

Psychic Treatment.—A simple life with as much rest as possible. The ideal would be to live in a crystal sphere, so as to be beyond all the jolts of a complicated life ; " Hide thy life," said Epicurus. " Simplify it to the maximum," said Tolstoy. It is evident that possessing these mottoes one can live in peace. These conditions, however, can scarcely be obtained outside of a sanatorium. " Carpe diem," said Horace. " Enjoy to-day as it comes, don't worry about to-morrow," and in this connection I recall that the distant view of events is like that of hills : when seen from a distance they seem so steep, but they flatten out as one gets nearer.

Neurological Treatment.—It is remarkable to note the considerable sensitiveness of these patients, and especially the frequency of headaches. An interesting point is that often they cannot go in electric tramways, because they get a headache as soon as they smell the ozone ; they also suffer from changes in atmospheric electrical tension ; this is why open flat country does not agree with them at first. They have, in an extraordinary degree, what my colleague and friend Sardou has called *meteorological sensibility*. These women can tell it is going to snow several days before it does, as æsthesiometers they are much more delicate than those one can buy.

Owing to the ease with which they tire themselves, one should order them only moderate exercise in carefully graduated amounts. There is one therapeutic measure which, neurologically, may be indicated—ultra-violet rays, for, due to their ability to fix calcium, these rays diminish the excitability of the vagus, and consequently the cenesthetic state and the oculo-cardiac reflex. But one must remember that these patients being hyper-cenesthetic, the dose must be infinitely less than for normal people. These cases, who the greater part of the time were considered by the old clinicians as hypochondriac, have indeed reactions out of all proportion to the quantities of stimulants applied.

From the endocrine point of view, one must reach the particular gland affected, and in the very first place attention should be given to any adrenal insufficiency, being very much on one's guard, if one is using opothera-peutic injections that one does not cause trouble, for these substances provoke very important vaso-motor reactions ; one must then use other substances that will have the desired effect, and the exhibition should be for long periods.

Now we have, in whole gland extract of pituitary, a remarkable preparation, which gives excellent results.

In addition there is ovarian treatment. One must, in these cases, try to calm down the hyperovarianism, whose significance we have seen. This can be done in two ways : either by marriage, or by drugs, of which the best is androstine, which I often use with great advantage.

In further endocrine treatment, one must exercise

o

patience; one can give, for example, small doses of thyroid (Léopold Lévy) in dose of 1 mmgr., to increase the basal rate, lessen the hypothyroidism, and diminish the frequency of the paroxysmal reactional crises of hyper-thyroidism.

Then calcium should be given, as this affects the meta-bolism, regulates the nervous system, diminishes the vagus excitability, and plays an important part from the point of view of the concentration of the forces of the nervous system in their proper order.

The visceral treatment is often mechanical. It is evident that apparatus which overcomes ptosis, par-ticularly belts with pneumatic cushions, will suppress in part the excitation of the solar system, which results from the dragging due to the ptosis.

One must also establish a special regime to combat the digestive troubles; and, in addition, to diminish the visceral manifestations, one will have to employ treat-ment to combat the alkalosis. With this object a seaside cure is excellent and usually very successful with vago-tonics. Sympathicotonics, however, do not benefit at all from sea air, indeed it is very harmful to them. As I say, it is excellent for vagotonics, and under the influence of a sea cure one can note the re-establishment of the solar reflex.

The hereditary gouty tendency has also to be dealt with, and in this connection one must remember that hereditary vitiation is like creases in cloth, which, the longer they have been there, the harder are they to remove. A remarkable means of altering this hereditary soil is *crenotherapy*, or spa treatment, provided it is used very early, from child-hood even.

As for the syphilitic factor, I refer you to the chapter dealing with this, in M. Hutinel's excellent book on the " Hereditary-syphilitic soil."

Tuberculous manifestations must be looked for with the greatest care, whether they are hereditary or acquired for it is of great prognostic value, on account of the undernourishment of these people, which may also be due to tuberculosis.

I have thought it advisable to bring to your notice these somewhat special clinical types which, while they may not be very severe, at least deserve to be described and set apart from others.

X

GENERAL PRINCIPLES OF TREATMENT OF THE PSYCHONEUROTIC

I PROPOSE to give you the general principles underlying the treatment of the psychoneurotic. I shall first make a synthetic study of these principles in their main directing lines exclusively, and then I shall speak of the treatment of the psychoneurotic and not of the treatment of the psychoneuroses ; for there is no treatment of the psychoneuroses. Landouzy used to insist on this—there is no morbid entity, hence no corresponding treatment.

Two great principles must be inscribed at the beginning of this subject.

1. The psychoneuroses being psycho-organic complexes, all standard symptomatic treatment is bad.

2. There is not a corresponding treatment for each symptom, but certain general conditions by their influence facilitate treatment as much as is possible.

Consequently, to treat the psychoneurotic with success, it is necessary not merely to have the necessary knowledge and touch, but it is also necessary that the patients should be in adequate surroundings.

I shall first deal with the *therapeutic environment*, before dealing with the *psychotherapy*, then I shall consider the adequate treatment in each zone that should be studied in the psychoneurotic—psychic zone, neurological zone, endocrine zone, visceral zone, and finally the morbific kernel.

I

THE THERAPEUTIC ENVIRONMENT

The ideal therapeutic environment is, for a great number of these cases, the sanatorium. It is evident that there are many psychoneurotics who cannot be cared for outside the sanatorium.

The advantages of the sanatorium are of three kinds :

1. First the *separation from the family*. If so many physicians, of great diagnostic and therapeutic ability, fail with psychoneurotic cases, it is because their influence is counteracted by the patient's family, even when the latter are very well disposed to the treatment. The psychoneurotic are not isolated peaks standing up above a plain ; usually they are merely summits which overtop surrounding heights. This is why Séglas often used to say to me : " When you arrive in a home, it is not always the person you have been called to see who is the sickest." One must get to know these families of neuropaths, of which the psychoneurotic are part, and the best service one can render them is to separate them from their surroundings.

I showed, in connection with the study of the psychic zone, the considerable influence of interpsychological relationships, on which Dupré rightly laid stress. This interpsychology puts a camouflage on the appearance of the patient, which one must in a fashion wash off to appreciate his true aspect.

Besides which, this separation of the patient from his family has not only got the negative advantage of getting him out of his surroundings ; it has this positive advantage—the legitimate wish of the patient, when his family is pleasant, to be able to return to it in the least possible time. There is no better way of activating the will to get well than this laudable desire to shorten as far as possible the stay in the sanatorium. The psychoneurotic can thus use his will to becoming well enough to get out of the institution where he has been sent.

2. In the second place comes the rôle of *talks*. This is a factor of great value, which enables us to communicate with others, only however up to a certain point. By conversation in a consulting-room one can only succeed in entering into the personality of the patient, in an incomplete fashion.

3. The third and much more important advantage is the opportunity it gives of studying the *general conduct* of the patient which the Anglo-Saxons call the *behaviour*. An illustrative proof of this is that intelligent families, before concluding an arrangement of marriage, often send the young couple on an engagement trip rather than on a wedding trip. There is no better way of getting to know the qualities and defects of character than sending the young man and woman travelling together. It is the conduct which is important, not the more or less marked camouflage of conversation between two people, such as takes place in a consulting-room, in which there are often grossly artificial elements.

For these reasons, then, in the sanatorium one is able to study methodically, regularly and daily, not only the conduct, but the general state, appetite, sleep, and activity of the person under observation. So that the sanatorium, provided it has a good and not too numerous medical staff, collaborators capable of noting a number of details, which the physician in charge cannot always be observing, is the ideal for the treatment of the psychoneurotic. It was for this reason that Gilbert Ballet, in his psychoneurotic service at the Hotel Dieu Hospital, had the nurses and the guard keep a book of " remarks," which very often was superior, from the documentary point of view, to the observations of the medical student-clerks. This was because the nurses, without worrying at all about the medical aspect, merely noted what they saw, whereas very often medical education seemed to interpose like a filter between the actuality and the observation made. The student is too apt to want to classify in small ready-made pigeonholes the observations he makes.

These are the advantages of the sanatorium, provided it is well situated. It should be wherever practicable in the country, and from the point of view of management, it should be large, commodious, airy and cheerful, with good light, sun and trees. Climate is a very important question, for as Landouzy used to say, " Health comes also by the eyes." In the second place, the success of the sanatorium must not be allowed to injure its doing good work. If there are too many patients and too few doctors, if enough time cannot be given to each case, the result is bad. The psychoneurotic needs to expand at ease with his doctor, so the latter must never seem to be in a hurry. It is bad to surround oneself with helpers who " fuss." In a sanatorium, in the case of the psychoneurotic as in other patients, the furtive gesture of the doctor who looks at his watch, has a very disagreeable effect on the patient. The physician must talk to the patient about his illness, must ask him about manifestations occurring both at night and by day. He must not, as some do, talk of irrelevant matters such as the stock market, politics, etc. No. With psychoneurotics the doctor must talk about the patient himself. If the latter wants to talk of something apart from himself well and good, but that should come little by little and not *proprio motu*.

The sanatorium should also be well equipped both medically and therapeutically, for the treatment of psychoneurotics is not merely a question of *psychotherapy*. There must also be *physiotherapy*. There must be a modern installation for exercises. It must be completely organized for physiotherapy, hydrotherapeutic, electrotherapeutic and X-rays. It is a question of doing things well, keeping in mind that often these therapeutic measures of a physical nature are only *methods of wrapping up psychotherapy*.

Psychotherapy is such an important branch of treatment that it is present in every prescription and very often the medicament becomes of value chiefly by the manner in which it is given—like charity.

Succedaneous to the sanatorium, there are other procedures that can and ought to be used.

Unfortunately, under present conditions in France, there is a very wide gap which exists to less degree in foreign countries. The good condition of the surroundings of the psychoneurotic are subordinate to financial considerations. For long, there was the belief that the psychoneurotic were all people of fortune, and that such cases did not occur among the poor. This is a mistake. They are found in all ranks of society, without taking into account that owing to the war many people have changed position and from this fact there has been a marked increase in their nervous reactions, thus one finds oneself in the unhappy position of seeing patients who are interesting from every point of view whom one cannot treat because they cannot afford sanatorium care. Now, in this connection hospital aid is inadequate—in a way there isn't any. Certainly at the St. Anne Hospital there is Dr. Toulouse's service, which in a way is the antechamber of the asylums, but if it does manage to do the work with its budget of a few hundred thousand francs a year, it is the only one that does so in the Seine Department.

I have certainly started here, at the Pitié Hospital, a small service for psychoneurotics, but I have absolutely no special facilities. I have no funds to carry it on : everything is lacking except the willingness of my loyal assistants. This lack is due to the Assistance publique, which in the present circumstances has done nothing adequate to ensure proper treatment of psychoneurotics, who are as interesting and even more so than the tuberculous, for the reason that, even though they are for the moment socially ineffective, with suitable treatment, they could quickly regain their physical and mental activity. Not only so, but they are people who are capable of producing intellectual work of social importance ; there would thus be the advantage, even financially, in providing them with proper treatment, but their condition makes less appeal than that of the tuberculous. The same campaigns have not been made on their behalf that have been made for the tuberculous, so that millions are being spent on people who are for the greater part of the time a net loss to the community, while for these others, who could be readily helped to recovery, absolutely nothing is done !

What is to be done about it ? The problem must be viewed from three aspects. First, certain parts of the services should be set aside to care for the psychoneurotic. These patients are not psychopaths who are unaware of their condition. Nor are they the acutely maniacal, for whom small isolation services have been set aside in most hospitals. There is no connection between them. The psychoneurotic are merely the simple depressed neurasthenics, who are cured by a stay of a few weeks in an adequate service. A big effort should therefore be made on their behalf, to provide hospitals, rooms, recreation rooms, such as are at their disposal in sanatoria. In Germany they take both rich and poor cases in the same institutions ; the same sanatorium for nervous diseases admits the patient who can pay 100 francs a day and the one who can pay nothing ; the comfort of the room is the only difference. I have just come from Barcelona, where the same system is in vogue, where in the same sanatorium, some patients pay 200 pesetas, and others five or six. The same scale should be in force here in Paris. And it is necessary to have more than just rooms and recreation rooms ; there should be physiotherapeutic installations near the patients' rooms, so that they do not have to go from one end of the building to the other for their treatment, for it is doubtful whether the fatigue of going and returning does not express itself algebraically as fatigue, destroying the good effects of hydrotherapy and physiotherapy.

But this is but one leg of the tripod of the treatment ; the second indispensable, whose lack I daily regret, is the *convalescent home* for the *after-cure* of these cases. The great majority of them, indeed, need a treatment which lasts some little time, but what is chiefly necessary, is that they should not have the feeling, which is so painful for them, that they may have to face again, from *one day to the next*, their daily life which they have already found so hard. It is for this reason that many of them relapse— as a refuge. The change should be a gradual one ; the necessity of the after-cure is a point on which Landouzy laid stress, and mineral water therapy is also an essential. What is needed is a Chateau somewhere just outside Paris. When we get such institutions organized, I am convinced that the results will be very much better.

In the third place, there is a need of the establishment for the psychoneurotic, what has been done for the tuberculous, in a certain number of general medical services and in children's services thanks to my friend Guinon, and which has not so far been done for nervous cases : I refer to " l'Œuvre sociale " and " l'Aide sociale " (Social Welfare Clinics). These are necessary to give these patients good advice on how to direct their hygiene, when they have been discharged from hospital, and also to advise their families. L'Aide sociale is as necessary here as it is for the tuberculous and for children.

When this threefold instrument is a fact the Assistance publique will have done a great service to Paris.

Houses of Retreat are also of great service. It is obvious that *æsthetic retreats* which can be established in certain artistic centres or in country of appropriate beauty, where establishments for æsthetic cures have been organized, would give great benefit. It is long since that the Catholic Church solved this question in the form of retreats in convents. It is beyond all doubt that for believers or for those who are not hostile to religion, a stay in a convent or in the sick houses attached to such institutions, is of great service in many cases. And I ought to say that, in view of life's difficulties, there are now a certain number of communities who have understood the importance of this way of looking at things, and have set apart several rooms where, in an atmosphere of religious calm, and for a moderate sum, a certain number of the depressed and psychoneurotic can complete their cure. Obviously one must not send there people suffering from scrupulous or contrast obsessions ; but on condition that the cases are suitably selected, it is certain that one may find in such institutions the halfway house between the sanatorium and the hospital, and for a price which is in some cases extremely modest.

Next comes the question of *travel*. Certainly some psychoneurotics may derive great benefit from travelling, which is for them a distraction, on the condition that it be done in comfort and without too frequent change from one place to another.

There is one form of it, which eliminates hotels, motor cars, and railways, and which is of enormous benefit to psychoneurotics—I mean *sea voyages*. They are especially suitable for the depressed, on whom the sea air has a very beneficial effect.

I come now to spas and mountain resorts.

It is beyond doubt that the climatic cure, on condition that the climate is suitably chosen, whether it be a seaside, mountain or plain resort, according to how it is sheltered from the wind, the degree of electrical tension of the atmosphere, is indicated for certain classes of case, and that the scale of climates is as extensive as the scale of types of psychoneurotics.

In the same way, there is a variety of spas suitable for different classes of psychoneurotics which are most useful.

I come now to *psychotherapy*. This is the therapy of the soul by means of psychic procedures, or at least chiefly so. It is very complex and to arrange it in order, I shall first consider psychotherapy in general, before studying the psychotherapy of the various types of psychoneurotics in particular.

1. *General Psychotherapy* must be divided into three great varieties according to whether one deals chiefly with the surface psychotherapy, which is applied to consciousness, or, on the other hand, the psychotherapy of the unconscious self, or, whether, being sufficiently synthetic, one is capable of viewing the whole ψυχή in its entirety, and deals with consciousness at the same time as with the unconscious self.

(*a*) *Superficial Psychotherapy.*—There is a superficial psychotherapy, which one cannot too strongly condemn, for it is invalid unless the personality of the psychologist is very great and acts on his patient by its prestige, in an indirect manner, and is independent of what he says to his patient. The first real superficial psychotherapy is the *rational psychotherapy*, which appeals exclusively to the reason and uses arguments in the form of syllogisms ; it is completely inadequate, for although reason is an excellent instrument with which to penetrate the complexity of the phenomena and from them deduce scientific laws, it is unable to modify the psychoneurotic disturbances, which are dependent chiefly on disturbances of instinct and cenesthesia, and which are only the expression of deeper disturbances of the organism. Thus it is an inadequate method, which however is sometimes useful to enhance and embody a more complex method.

(*b*) *Affective Psychotherapy* is the second form of superficial psychotherapy. It is what the family does spontaneously to the patient. It is inadequate and sometimes very dangerous. It is done in two ways, first in the form of an excessive interest, and a tearful sympathy, which only aggravate the neuropathic manifestations and sometimes cause fresh ones to appear. This is how one sees many cases of depression complicated by hysterical manifestations due to the family's influence. Or it may take the form of affective therapeusis by reprimands ; when the family reproach the patient with being ill only in imagination—with lacking will-power. This attitude only makes the condition of these wretched psychoneurotics worse. In this direction the physician may be extremely useful in getting the patients to understand that their state is no exceptional one, that their troubles are not unusual, that they are in the nature of an illness like any other trouble, and above all that they are not imaginary, and this is my attitude in such cases to the family.

I say : The parents or the husband must have a sympathetic attitude towards the patient, then they must raise the patient's morale by telling her not to worry, for the trouble is merely superficial, etc. ; thus, on the one hand, affective attitude sympathetic, but on the other a firm rational attitude, of confidence and hope for a speedy recovery.

2. *Psychotherapy of the Unconscious Self.*

In the psychotherapy of the unconscious self two main systems with the superaddition of mysticism are to be distinguished. First, empirical methods ; and second, the more recent symptomatic methods in the perhaps somewhat overdone manner of Freud.

The empirical type of psychotherapy of the unconscious self with superadded mysticism goes back almost to the origin of man. I shall not here go into the study of this form of oriental civilization, in India. It is evident that the most perfect form of empirical psychotherapy of the unconscious self was already practised by the priests of Æsculapius in the great temple of Epidaurus. A remarkable lecture has recently been given by Prof. Vaquez on his return from Greece. He gave a very clear account of their psychotherapeutic cure of the unconscious self. It was mainly a question of *onirotherapy*. You know that the sick entered the temple after fumigating and purifying themselves with a mixture of aromatic plants and incense. They lay down under the portico and went to sleep, dreaming all kinds of dreams, and passed the night there. Next day the priest questioned them about their dreams and prescribed treatment according to the dreams given. He found thus in these dreams the crystallized morbific kernel enabling him to make suggestions. The results obtained by the psychotherapy of Epidaurus were so famous that this temple became the centre of a great pilgrimage of both Greeks and Barbarians, who came for treatment.

This tradition became lost little by little, but it was reborn in another form with the development of Christianity during the Middle Ages. And I shall recall to your minds the exorcisms which played a very important part then. They exist even up to this day and psychotherapeutic exorcisms still are successful with some patients.

Then there are corrupt forms of these religious procedures which merge into magic. Magic, which has been the origin of psychology, has continued to play a part in psychotherapy, and in certain cases the magical proceedings of sympathetic magic are not always completely lacking in social usefulness. This is a point on which I laid stress, at the Pinel centenary, in connection with the case of Barbiguier.[1] This was a patient who had a systematized interpretative insanity. He had the firm conviction that he was persecuted by evil sprites. These took the form of a number of people, even the shape of the great Pinel himself, and Barbiguier had hit upon a means of ridding himself of these tormenting spirits. He made a small statue in the semblance of the incarnation of the spirit which obsessed him and pricked it with a pin. While he did so, he did not have any wish to attack the person with a weapon.

It was certainly, from the social point of view, an excellent substitute, for instead of murdering the enemies who pursued him, he was satisfied with pricking their incarnated image with a pin. This is a most useful application of magic, in a way beneficial to public welfare. But this did not in any way have any scientific quality. It became necessary, at the time when the Encyclopædia

---

[1] Laignel-Lavastine et Jean Vinchon, *Deux malades de Pinel*; Barbiguier et Martin de Gallardon. *Congrès de aliénists et neurologists*, Genève-Lausanne, Aug., 1926.

(of Alembert & Diderot) was dominating the field, to colour psychotherapy a scientific tint, and thus it was that magnetism was born with Mesmer's vat. It afterwards lost its theatrical trappings and became reduced to hypnotism. The question then arose whether the patient was suggestible because he was in hypnosis, or whether he was hypnotized because he had received suggestions. Babinski has shown that hypnosis is a function of the suggestibility of the individual, which indeed varies in different people. Certainly, from the point of view of psychotherapy of the unconscious self, the best way of using it, is oftenest as *hetero-suggestion.* You know what we owe to Bernheim in the development of hetero-suggestion and the means physicians employ, many of which are empirical, to assist the therapeutic ideas, which they want to use, to actively penetrate into the unconscious self of the patient. It is in this that there lies the cardinal difference between persuasion and suggestion. Suggestion is the entry, by breaking in, of feelings or wishes, into the unconscious self of the individual, which one wants to reach there.

Besides this there are forms of hetero-suggestion, which have come to assume a great importance, in a religious form, and which, if carried to excess, may be really dangerous from the social aspect. In this connection I should like to say a word on the subject of " Christian Science." This consists in a systematization, on a religious basis, of hetero-suggestion, which in many cases is extremely useful. There are many Christian scientists who successfully cure patients, but where they overdo it is when they oppose their patients attending a physician. This is a true abuse of the legal practice of medicine. For in cases of infectious or organic diseases, in which serotherapy is essential, the Christian scientist may be the cause of criminally allowing people to die.

The latest method of applying suggestion, which has recently had a great vogue and is still growing, in spite of the fact that its initiator is now dead, is an auto-suggestion, which consists of reciting simple formulæ at different times of the day, such as those used by the pharmacist Coué, who advised people to repeat morning and evening, for example, " Every day, in every way, I get better and better ! "

From the empirical standpoint, there are not only those manifestations, where the element of suggestion is obvious, but there are also cures whose mechanism is obscure, and in which an element of suggestion cannot be denied. Such are the religious cures, and there is in France a great religious centre of this sort, where many cures are observed—I refer to Lourdes. At Lourdes, the cures are of a variety of kinds, but there are certainly some of them which interest us here, that is they are due to a process of suggestion. I don't want to labour this point, I merely wish to remark that in certain cases there is absolutely no doubt that there is an element of suggestion in the recovery. And further these are the cases which are not recorded by the Bureau of Records (Bureau des Constatations).

Apart from empirical uses the *Systematic Method* has to be considered. It is a method, which at present seems to become world-wide, like an epidemic, and which is ravaging chiefly the Anglo-Saxon peoples and the peoples amongst whom Catholicism is not dominant. It is noteworthy that Freudian psychoanalysis is an " ersatz " confession, and that those peoples who have retained Catholic confession are less inclined to be carried away by the psychoanalytic method. Psychoanalysis, as established by Freud, is of service, but it is by no means a new thing. It was at the Saltpêtrière that Freud did his first researches, and in this he only followed the teaching of my master Pierre Janet, who was then already studying the effects of repression and was using the psychotherapy of the unconscious self. But French psychology demands qualities of finesse in the various individual procedures of each case, which is an enormous hygienic labour. On the contrary the Freudist psychoanalysis standardizes, it is a psychotherapy " omnibus," a psychotherapy of the novelty shops, on hand for the first doctor who comes along, who may have no special knowledge, and this is why this method, which belongs strictly to the medical field, is exploited by a number of people, philosophers, Protestant ministers, masseurs, etc., who have no knowledge of medicine. This is a great disadvantage. This was why when psychoanalysis was up for discussion at the Besançon Congress, I thought it necessary to draw a distinction between the Freudism of the Freudian and that of the Freudists.

Freudism is a doctrine which begins with a technique and ends in systematized conclusions. The *Freudians* are the frequently very remarkably intelligent disciples of Freud, who make very interesting studies on the relationships between the prelogical psychoanalysis and the origin of myths ; and lastly the *Freudists*, the empiricists who take only the systematized side of the doctrine, who are content with simple formulæ instead of understanding the substance, and, in short, fly to extremes which are dangerous for the patients.

II

After this review of General Psychotherapy, both of the superficial and the unconscious aspects, I come now to the study of the best method, which is the synthetic method of my master Pierre Janet, which he exposed in full in his three volumes of " Medications psychologiques," published in 1924 by Alcan, in which he indicates the method of purgation, in which the individual rids himself of all the contingencies, all the complications of his existence, which method tends to simplification, recalling the maxim of Epicurus, when he said : " Hide thy life," and that of Tolstoy : " Simplify your life to the maximum."

I come now to the study of the sublimation of tendencies. The tendencies can be divided into three categories.

P

The *Lower Tendencies* which are characterized by the interpretation put on cenesthesia; the *Higher Tendencies* characterised by synthetically produced high ideals, moral or religious; and the *Intermediate Tendencies,* characterized on the one hand by their goal, which is a higher synthetic aim, and on the other hand by their origin, which is local, cenesthetic.

It is chiefly these intermediate tendencies which characterize the psychoneurotic; consequently the objective of this second part of synthetic psychotherapy consists in knowing how to "sublimate" the intermediate tendencies in order to guide them towards the higher tendencies. This *sublimation* is in a way the important process in education, granted that we are *a bundle of instincts bound together by the higher synthetic functions* and all civilization and the education of oneself consists in learning to sublimate these instincts, so that they may blossom out as moral, religious, or social flowers, instead of achieving only an elementary reflex derived from the surge of primitive instinct.

Psychotherapy of the forms of neuroses in themselves.— These are simply the application of the foregoing principles to the particular reactions which each psychoneurotic may present at certain times.

A word on the psychotherapy applied to *hysterical, neurasthenic, obsessive,* and *hyperemotive manifestations.*

Reference the *hysterical cases* : there is a basic principle which must always be kept in mind, it is this, that, the hysterical being like children, the will-power of their physician must always dominate them in a way like a sword of Damocles. Let us never promise to a hysterical patient something we cannot carry out, for, if one deceives him or lets him down, all is lost.

What degree of severe psychotherapy may one apply to the hysterical ? This is a delicate question. The question of importance is not the form of the reactions occurring in the patient, so much as the underlying character of the patient showing the reactions. One must therefore *study the character of the patient* before one can tell whether one can get results by gentle methods, or whether it will be necessary to employ severe methods. I must admit that often one is obliged to have recourse to severe methods consisting in using more or less strong electric currents, which may go as far as to produce shock, such as we used during the war, so severe as to be painful, but which by the psychic revulsion which it provokes, causes the disappearance of excessive symptoms. It is certain that a large number of hysterical crises are cured by severe methods.

Sometimes a simple change in regime, complete isolation, gives satisfactory results, but in severe cases one should not hesitate to use powerful convulsing electric currents. Sometimes one must obtain the patient's co-operation and not hesitate to get him to promise in writing that up to a certain date he will have no further manifestations, failing which there will be the penalty of something for which he may happen to have a particular dislike. These patients may sometimes be very troublesome, and, if in some cases one has success from the start, in others many difficulties arise. In such cases one must not hesitate to change the treatment for a more vigorous one.

The chronic manifestations of hysteria are sometimes easier to cure than the paroxysmal ones, especially if the patients come to one from a distance, if they have had trouble in getting themselves cared for by the physician, and so have had the time to crystallize their wishes on him from whom they hope to obtain a cure.

Thus in the case of a young servant, who had seen her mistress fall into a pool, and who had been so upset by this that she had felt her legs give way beneath her and her voice fail her, as the poet has it : " vox faucibus haesit." She thereafter was confined to bed at home, the centre of a great popular interest. She had had 800 injections of morphine, and had been seen by some sixty physicians. For ten years she had been an immobile bedridden incurable, who never spoke, but who had always been occupied with some form of work. She had no money, and to get into hospital she had to pay a month in advance, for the "Assistance publique" does not provide for hospital cases who are strangers to the locality. After negotiations, which lasted some five or six weeks, she was at last admitted to my service. Thus, as a physician, I had the prestige of distance and of being difficult of access. This is of great importance. I made her sit down in front of me, and made her say 1, 2, 3, 4, 5, 6 ; at the end of five minutes she spoke. Then I worked on her legs and she moved them ; next day I continued these exercises and in three days' time she was cured. It was a splendid result, and the patient made a triumphant return to her own district.

One form, which ordinarily does very well in the sanatorium, but which is very serious and may terminate fatally if it is not treated properly, is *Mental Anorexia*. It is one of the crowning successes of psychotherapy. There was a case of a young girl, 160 cms. in height and weighing 30 kilos. ; thin as a skeleton, she was believed to have tuberculosis. She was first put to bed and psychotherapy begun. This consisted in making her take regularly a certain amount of food ; she pretended she could not swallow ; but she could, perfectly well. She was persuaded to do so, and in the end she put on three kilos per week. But one must be on one's guard for the ruses employed by such cases of mental anorexia. They endeavour to deceive one by all sorts of means : she tried to vomit, for example. Then it is necessary to find the reasons which have driven her to this anorexia. These are multiple ; very often because the young girl—it is always a question of young women—is sometimes somewhat stout ; or sometimes because their familial situation drives them to do nothing ; in short, one must try to get to the bottom of the trouble. But, I repeat, psychotherapy in such cases, when applied outside the sphere of familial influence, gives marvellous results.

Special Treatment of the Neurasthenic Form.—The chief means in this form is the Weir Mitchell treatment, that is to say, rest in bed, for the dominant factor in these cases is fatigue. They therefore need absolute rest and quiet. Sleep then returns little by little, as does also the appetite, then they gain a little in weight. But sometimes there is present in these cases a state of auto-suggestion which comes from the fear they have of having a series of illnesses, a fear which can disappear entirely from the mind of the hypochondriac who asks for nothing better than to be rid of it.

I emphasize therefore these two cardinal points. Treat the fatigue ; and treat the auto-suggestive state which is related to the fear of a series of illnesses.

The proper treatment of the *Obsessed* is a much more delicate matter, and it is here that the Freudian psychoanalysis is of use in showing where the psychic trauma originates, sometimes going as far back as childhood, or arising in an affective complex which the patient carefully hides. When this has been laid bare the obsessed patient is eased and rid of it.

Amongst the obsessed, there is a certain number that one might call the *psychoanalytic neurotics*. In such, there is first a history of a genital source of their trouble, which has been lost from consciousness, but which still continues to play an important part in the unconscious self, and one does not successfully cure the patient until one has got to the bottom of all this story. Such is the very particular psychoanalytic form with illness of a genital or religious origin, in which it is absolutely necessary to have recourse to Freudian psychology to clean up the mental state of the patient.

At the same time there is usually paroxysmal predominance of obsession related to some state of depression. This depression must be attended to, anxiety must be allayed, the vagotonia, which is usually present in such cases, must be combated, and an attempt should be made to see if, by the dream cathartic method, which is often very important in the obsessed, one can place the personality on the right line. There is, indeed, a symbolism, which exists in the depths of the being, and it appears likely that, in many cases, the dream may be the symbolization of a wish and that, when these patients have realized their wishes through the symbolism of their dreams, they may be rid of these wishes in their daily behaviour. One might thus say "happy are the dreamers, who thus rid themselves, in their dreams, without danger to society of their anti-social impulses or desires ! " There is thus the advantage, in the psychoneurotic, of being able to develop their dreams, so that they may rid themselves of their troublesome tendencies.

Certain substances help in the attainment of this effect : for example, opium, laudanum, which, in some cases aids in the production of a richer *dream flowering*, which is generally of the opposite colour to that which is dominant in the waking state. In this way one may be very much impressed, in cases of anxiety-melancholia, with the good effects of treatment by laudanum. I shall leave it at that.

Lastly, in connection with the *Hyperemotive*, one may say that the thing which marks the quality of the physician, is not so much what he says, as what he does not say. Weigh all your words, for with these hyperemotive, disturbed people, the least word may be the cause of extremely dangerous trains of thought, and with a misunderstood word one may undo all the good that has already begun after one or two weeks of psychotherapy. Such are the general principles governing the treatment of the psychoneurotic. They form the basis on which is built the adequate therapeusis of each zone that has to be studied in these patients: the psychic zone, the nervous zone, the endocrine zone, and lastly the morbific kernel.

INDEX

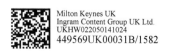